Osteopathic Medicine in Oregon

A Look Back

Osteopathic Medicine in Oregon

A Look Back

Best Wishes as you begin your studies
to become a D.O.

John Stiger, DO

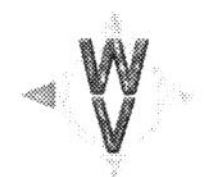

WestView Publishing
Mount Vernon, Washington

Cover design: Rylan Schubkegel
Interior design: Diane Johnson, PageCraft
Text Editor: Diane Johnson, PageCraft

ISBN: 978-0-9863258-0-9

Library of Congress Control Number: 2014960004

Published by
WestView Publishing
Mount Vernon, Washington

Printed in the United States of America

This book is dedicated to:

The wonderful osteopathic physicians and educators
at my alma mater, Chicago College of Osteopathic Medicine;
my colleagues and mentors at Eastmoreland Hospital;
and John Bauers, DO, who took a young DO under his wing,
first as an associate and later as a partner in the practice
he established in Oak Grove, Oregon.

Table of Contents

Section Five: The People

Foreword

It has been my pleasure to have been mentored by and worked beside John Stiger, DO, for many years. When he began this project of recounting the history of our great profession in the state of Oregon, I had no idea he would honor me by requesting that I contribute to it with a foreword. This will be brief as it should not detract from his fine work.

Dr. Stiger takes us through the early days of osteopathic medicine as it evolved from the allopathic world. We see how it struggled for identity and recognition and then changed again to be become more traditional, yet different. Dr. Stiger captures this struggle for acceptance as he tours us through the 20th century, culminating in the development of a bright new osteopathic medical school in Lebanon, Oregon. We learn of those who brought the osteopathic profession to its present status in Oregon and recognize how exciting the future can be for these young physicians being trained in the state-of-the-art building by a remarkable team of physicians and basic science faculty.

Osteopathic physicians should stand tall as they look at the present and future of this rapidly growing profession. There are now over thirty osteopathic medical schools across the country and DOs comprise twenty percent of the graduation doctors each year.

When COMP-Northwest graduates its first class of 105 students in June 2015, it will join the 225 graduating from the Pomona campus, for a total of 330 graduates. This will make the Western University of Health Science and its osteopathic medical schools—COMP and COMP-Northwest—one of the largest graduating medical school classes in the country. In this constantly evolving world of health care, the osteopathic profession is proving to be part of the solution and not part of the problem.

Thank you, Dr. John Stiger, for your excellent rendition of a tumultuous time for a proud profession. We are forever in your debt.

Your humble colleague and student,

Paula M. Crone, DO
Dean of COMP and COMP-Northwest
November, 2014

Preface

On Saturday August 5, 2012, I was seated on the podium of the church auditorium where the second "white coat" ceremony was held at the College of Osteopathic Medicine of the Pacific Northwest (COMP-Northwest), the new osteopathic medical school in Lebanon, Oregon. As I listened to the speakers I couldn't help but marvel that there even was an osteopathic medical school in Oregon, much less located in a small rural town like Lebanon! How did this all come about? What was the chain of events that led up to this moment?

I am a retired osteopathic general practitioner. After serving a rotating internship at Eastmoreland General Hospital in Portland, Oregon, I was offered a position by John Bauers, DO. Bauers, a graduate of the Kansas City College of Osteopathic Medicine, had also interned at Eastmoreland Hospital, known at the time as Portland Osteopathic Hospital. He had established a very successful practice in Oak Grove, a small suburb of Portland. In 1974, I joined Bauers as a partner and, after his retirement, continued at that location until my retirement in 2008.

When I entered practice, my entire focus was to be a competent, successful doctor who was respected in the community and by my colleagues. Although I was active on the staff of Eastmoreland Hospital, in the Osteopathic Foundation, and in the Osteopathic

Association, I had only a vague understanding of the history of the profession in the Oregon.

Upon retiring I decided to learn more. I started by interviewing every "old timer" I could locate. Sometimes it was the spouse or friends or the family of the doctor; on occasion it was the retired doctor him- or herself. (I quickly learned that the interviews with the doctors were far more productive if the spouse of the doctor participated.) With every interview, I learned more about the history of the profession in Oregon, great personal stories about the doctors I interviewed, and the names of other DOs of whom I had never heard.

It has been a thoroughly enjoyable enterprise. All of these doctors shared common traits: they were hard working, dedicated, and have had such interesting careers! Some have city parks dedicated to them; some have spots in local museums dedicated to their personal history. Most practiced in smaller towns where they had important roles to play, not only as physicians but also as local school board members, team doctors for schools, and active members in groups like Rotary, Kiwanis, and Scouting. Most were active in their local churches, where they served as deacons or board members. They advised local fire departments, trained volunteers in first aid, and served as county coroners or on the Board of Medical Examiners.

Their caring attitude toward their patients and the use of osteopathic methods endeared them to their patients. The testimonies and efforts of these loyal patients were instrumental in helping to pass legislation in the state legislature, often in the face of strong and unrelenting opposition by the allopathic profession.

At first I considered blogging these essays, but I quickly realized I didn't even know what a blog was. I had lunch with Dave Walls, executive secretary of our state osteopathic association, the Osteopathic Physicians and Surgeons of Oregon (OPSO), who kindly suggested they be posted on the association's website. As the essays accumulated, I realized that a book would be inevitable.

These oral histories were wonderful, but they really didn't provide much information about what had transpired prior to 1940. I contacted Kathleen Haley of the Oregon Medical Board and asked if there was a list of all of the DOs that had been licensed in the state since 1900. Yes, there probably was such a list in the archives in Salem; most of that material has never been digitized. However, she did forward a list of sixty-seven DOs that were licensed on the same day in January of 1908; thirty-five percent of these were women. There was no other information about these doctors except their names and the date of licensure.

At the time I was interviewing Rolland O'Dell, DO, a retired cardiologist, and his wife, Diane. I mentioned the list and Diane asked if she could do some research through her genealogy group. In a few days, she was able to obtain more information, much of it very interesting—but what did it mean?

Bill Bryon, PhD, a consultant for the COMP-Northwest, advised us to form a search committee. As members of the search committee, Diane O'Dell, Brian Walls, and I interviewed three research candidates from the history graduate school at Portland State University. We agreed that expertise in searching the web and young eyes to scrutinize the material were crucial, and we selected Rhiannon Orizaga, a master's candidate, to be our researcher. With a generous grant from OPSO, we tasked Rhiannon with learning more about the names on the 1908 list and as much as possible about the osteopathic profession in earlier times.

The first task was to read about the early history of the profession. Books and journals, both about the history of the osteopathic profession in general and the history of Oregon, were helpful in this research.

The first section of this book chronicles the life of A. T. Still, who renounced his MD training and embarked on a new concept he named osteopathic medicine.

The first graduates of American School of Osteopathy (ASO) came to Oregon in 1900, and we explore several questions in Chapter 2. What sort of challenges did these practitioners face in Oregon? Did the training they received at Kirksville prepare them adequately for these challenges? How were they received by the public and other doctors already practicing in the state? What sort of relationship did these early DOs have with the state legislature? What sorts of regulation or limitations were placed on the practice of osteopathic medicine in Oregon?

In subsequent chapters, we discuss the evolution of osteopathic medicine in the nation and in Oregon. We examine the tensions that arose between the traditionalists who continued to limit their practices to the classic methods taught by Still and the DOs who incorporated advances in medicine into their practices. We review how the training programs in the osteopathic medical schools slowly evolved, incorporating modern advances while preserving the osteopathic principles that have proven so successful.

By the 1940s, graduates of osteopathic medical schools were educated on a par with allopathic physicians, yet they continued to be barred from practice in large MD hospitals and the military. We discuss how the continuing opposition by the allopathic profession led to the advent of osteopathic hospitals in Oregon.

We will discuss the struggles of the osteopathic profession during the fight for equality, as well as the challenges facing the profession from the many cost containment efforts over the years, and the availability and spiraling cost of medical malpractice insurance.

We will also look at how the graduate and post-graduate education of osteopathic physicians has changed over the years. Due to the formation of a number of new osteopathic medical schools, the profession has reemerged as an important source of well-trained medical students who are prepared to serve as primary care doctors or as trainees in residency programs. Our new osteopathic medical school, COMP-Northwest in Lebanon, is an example.

Section One

The Beginnings of Osteopathy

CHAPTER 1

Advances in Medical Care 1850–1900

From the beginning of the nineteenth century, there was public dissatisfaction with and distrust of the medical practices of the time. The use of bleeding, purges, highly toxic medicines, and other methods horrified the public and prepared the way for "alternative" methods of treatment to develop.

One early example of these alternative methods was the Samuel Thompson (1769–1843) Method, which was based on the theory that the body needed a fever to rid itself of disease. Substances that induced a fever were administered to the patient, and, at the time, these were successful enough to allow this method to continue.[1]

Samuel Hahnemann (1755–1834) developed a method termed "homeopathy." This approach was based on the concept of administering a substance, called a homeopathic substance, whose side effects mimicked the symptoms of a specific disease. That disease was treated by administering minute quantities of the homeopathic substance. One example of such a substance was quinine. In large doses to the healthy individual, quinine produced symptoms of malaria, but in small amounts, it successfully treated the disease. Hahnemann used himself as a trial patient, testing over four hundred substances during his lifetime.[2] Hahnemann first coined the term "allopaths" to describe the medical doctors (MDs) of the time.

Homeopathy gained wide acceptance and today one can still find medical schools that were formerly homeopathic medical schools.[3] Some of these homeopathic substances have been incorporated into "naturopathy" and chiropractic. Since these substances usually come from natural plants, they are called "naturopathic" substances and are regulated by the Food and Drug Administration as food substances rather than medications.[4]

Another method, called "eclecticism," was developed by Wooster Beach (1794–1868). This approach drew from both homeopathy and the Thompson Method.[5] "Drugless therapies" were also in vogue at the time, including cold-water treatments, spa treatments (mineral waters), the Swedish Movement Method, and Mesmer's Magnetism Method. It has been estimated that nearly fifteen percent of the overall population were using these methods.

Practitioners of all these methods were called MDs, and many were licensed and practiced in Oregon.[6] Most of the MDs practicing in the western part of the United States would have received their training as apprentices to established physicians because all the actual medical schools were on the East Coast.[7]

Introducing Osteopathy

During this period, there emerged an interesting and charismatic figure who would make an important contribution to health care in the United States: Andrew Taylor (A. T.) Still, MD.

Still was born on August 6, 1828, in Jonesville, Virginia, the third of nine children. His father, Abram Still, MD, was an itinerant Methodist preacher, a farmer, and a doctor who had to support his large family in any way he could. As a Methodist missionary, Abram Still was constantly on the move as new towns sprang up in the West; these were fertile grounds for "revival" meetings leading to the establishment of new Methodist churches. Perhaps it was at these meetings that A. T. Still learned the art of public speaking and how to generate enthusiasm for a cause. Despite being on the road a great deal, Abram Still made sure that his children received the best education available.

In 1851, A. T. Still finished his education and settled down to become a farmer. After two years, he decided that farming was not for him, and he decided to become a doctor. He was invited to apprentice with his father, who was working as a doctor at the Wakarusa Indian Mission in Kansas. Under the guidance of his father, Still studied medicine and practiced by treating the Shawnee Indians who resided at the mission. He was keenly interested in anatomy, and he provided himself with anatomical specimens by making nighttime raids on the burial sites of Indians who were victims of a cholera epidemic raging through the Shawnee tribe at the time.[8]

By this time, the politics that would soon embroil the entire nation in a civil war were very much in evidence in the Kansas and Missouri territories. At issue was the dispute as to whether these future states would allow slavery. Still soon became involved in the controversy, forming a cadre of irregulars that was later incorporated into the Union army. While serving in the Union cavalry, he was nearly killed in the battle to repel a confederate invasion of Kansas City. He left the military in 1864 and returned to his farm to resume his career as an MD.[9]

A few months after returning to civilian life, tragedy struck. Despite the best efforts of his MD colleagues, three of his children died of meningitis. After witnessing firsthand the futility of the medical treatments of his children, he began to question the methods that he had been taught and to study alternative methods for treatment of disease. As he studied these methods, he realized that, in general, these alternative methods seemed to cause less harm to patients.

He gradually concluded that internal medication of any kind was invalid and probably immoral as well.[10] In 1874, Still renounced his MD degree and began to apply his own ideas of treatment, based largely on the concept that given good nutrition, proper hydration, massage, and rest, the human body could heal itself. The doctor's role was to educate and encourage patients so they were better able to recover. This apparently outraged the local doctors and community leaders, and soon he was expelled from the local Methodist church and scorned and ridiculed by the local MDs. Ostracized in Baldwin, Kansas, he moved to Macon, Missouri, where his ideas and methods were again scorned and ridiculed.[11]

In the 1870s, Still was exposed to and quickly learned the art of "bonesetting." This method of reducing dislocations and adjusting the spine had been known for hundreds of years. Still quickly became known as a "lightning bonesetter," and when he added bonesetting treatments to his other concepts, he began to experience some success.[12]

After relocating to Kirksville, Missouri, Still traveled to other towns where he demonstrated his skill as a bonesetter. A crowd would gather, and Still, standing on a platform formed by his horse-drawn wagon, would lecture a bit on his ideas. Then he would spot someone in the crowd who was having problems that might respond to bonesetting, and he would give a treatment on the spot.[13] He became so popular that he no longer had to travel to find patients; they would come to him in Kirksville.

By this time, Still had developed a unique philosophy of healing which he termed "osteopathy." He maintained that the human body had the intrinsic ability to heal itself, and that the use of medication was actually impeding the ability of the body in this healing process. It was the task of the osteopathic physician to identify, through observation and palpation, abnormalities of the spinal column and other parts of the body that impeded normal mechanical, circulatory, and sensory functions. Using osteopathic methods, the physician was often able to normalize these functions, enabling the body to return to its normal healthy state. Without any sort of medication, the combination of proper diet, hydration, abstinence from smoking and alcohol, rest, and manipulation produced remarkable successes.[14]

Still opened the American School of Osteopathy (ASO) in Kirksville in 1892. Tuition was $500. Classes started on October 3, 1892, with an initial student body of twenty-one men and women. The ages of the students ranged from eighteen to sixty-five, and their educational backgrounds varied as well. The common factor was that all of the students or members of the student's families had been successfully treated by Still.[15]

One of his first students was William Smith, an MD trained in Edinburgh, Scotland, and in continental Europe. At the time, Smith was in the employ of a surgical instrument company and happened to learn about Still from some of the local MDs, who labeled Still a "blankety-blank" quack. Curious, Smith looked up Still. He was so impressed by what Still was accomplishing that when he was offered training in Still's osteopathic methods in exchange for teaching anatomy at ASO, he accepted.[16]

The curriculum was arranged so that students studied anatomy in the mornings with Smith, then spent the afternoons with Still, "the old doctor," studying osteopathic concepts and methods in the infirmary located next door.

From 1892 to 1896, three classes graduated, with training lasting from nine to eighteen months. A bill introduced into the Missouri legislature in 1896 was written to grant full recognition and licensure to the osteopathic profession. The bill passed the legislature, but it was vetoed by the governor on the grounds that DOs were insufficiently trained to be granted full practice rights.[17]

This setback forced Still to expand the school curriculum beyond anatomy and osteopathic methods. He added physiology, surgery theory and practice, midwifery, toxicology, histology, urinalysis, pathology, and symptomology to the curriculum, and he hired faculty members to teach these topics. Still continued to be adamantly opposed to the subject "materia medica" and pharmacology, and these subjects were not included in the curriculum until he retired in 1918.[18]

The "old doctor," as he was called by his students, enjoyed having his picture taken. He would pose with his students clustered around a partially dissected cadaver, or in graduation pictures of the classes he trained. In practically every photo, he is dressed in a formal suit with vest and watch fob, knee high boots, and a broad-brimmed black hat. In one widely published pose, he is seated, a bearded, bespectacled man turned to the left as he peers intently at the femur he often carried with him. Presumably, he would lecture on anatomy or biomechanics using the femur to demonstrate. His rambling lecture style included philosophical observations and analogies to demonstrate his points.

A most unusual and charismatic doctor, this father of osteopathic medicine![19]

The Profession Grows

The osteopathic school, the associated clinics and infirmary, and the hospitals in Kirksville enjoyed great success. People literally flocked to Kirksville for treatments that would sometime last for weeks. While under care, these patients stayed in local hotels and frequented local restaurants and other businesses. Railroads added special trains that ran four times daily to accommodate the traffic of people coming to and from the Kirksville Osteopathic Clinic.[20]

Graduates of ASO were soon founding their own colleges of osteopathic medicine. Some of the first were National School of Osteopathy in Kansas City in 1895, and in 1896, Pacific College of Osteopathy in Los Angeles, Northern Institute of Osteopathic Medicine in Minneapolis, and Still College of Osteopathic Medicine in Des Moines. Schools appeared in other American cities including Boston; Chicago; Philadelphia; Wilkes Barre, Pennsylvania; Ottawa, Kansas; Franklin, Kentucky; Fargo, North Dakota; Keokuk, Iowa; and Quincy, Illinois. Initially the curriculum of the new schools closely resembled that of the parent school in Kirksville. In time, some of these schools prospered and endured, while others, such as the Northern Institute, were absorbed or closed.[21]

Graduates tended to locate their practices close to the school where they trained, often assisting in the training of the students that were following them. By 1904, an estimated four thousand DOs were in practice, and approximately half were graduates of these new schools.[22]

The training at some of these schools was marginal at best. The teaching staffs were small, generally between three and ten professors, depending on the size of the school. The instructors often did not possess DO degrees, but were MDs who desired to learn more about osteopathy. In exchange for their services, these teaching MDs were often awarded DO degrees in much less time than their fellow students. The facilities and equipment in these schools also varied widely, from large spacious facilities equipped with microscopes and X-ray equipment to schools with only a small room with a treatment table and wall charts.

Osteopathic medicine was promoted to prospective students as a way to earn a handsome income. Highly qualified women who were discouraged from applying to allopathic schools because of their gender found that they were welcomed at the osteopathic schools. By 1910, women formed approximately thirty-five percent of students studying osteopathic medicine.[23] These women osteopathic physicians were often at the top of their classes academically, and they subsequently made important contributions to the profession as physicians and as researchers.[24]

By 1900, some schools had become nothing more than "diploma mills." Schools such as Noe's College of Osteopathy in San Francisco, and Payne's College of Osteopathy and Optics in Ottawa, Kansas, among others, were issuing DO diplomas to anyone who could pay the fee. Recognizing the negative effect of these "mills" and the uneven quality of the education provided by some of the other schools, the American Osteopathic Association (AOA), established in 1901, formed a subcommittee called the Associated Colleges of Osteopathy (ACO). This committee developed standards of education for all osteopathic medical schools desiring accreditation by the AOA.[25]

There were 717 graduates from ASO in Kirksville by 1900. Seventeen percent located close to the school, eleven percent elsewhere in Missouri, twelve percent in Iowa, seven percent in Illinois, five percent in Ohio, and four percent in Pennsylvania and New York. The remaining graduates were scattered around the rest of the country. Some of these graduates were sponsored by wealthy clients who wished to continue the treatments begun in Kirksville. Other graduates returned to their hometowns to begin practice.[26]

In 1903, Eamons Booth, PhD, DO, a highly respected educator at Washington University in St. Louis, was hired to survey all of the existing osteopathic schools in the country. His report led to many changes in osteopathic education, including a compulsory three-year, twenty-seven month curriculum, which became official AOA policy in 1904. In 1910, Abraham Flexner, a graduate of Johns Hopkins and a medical educator, was retained by the Rockefeller Foundation to conduct a survey of all colleges of medicine, including osteopathic schools. His findings and recommendations paved the way for far higher standards in all medical schools across the country. As a result of the higher standards brought about by these two reports, by 1915 there were far fewer colleges of allopathic medicine, and only seven recognized colleges of osteopathic medicine remained.[27]

Early Challenges for Osteopathic Physicians

One of the many obstacles that the new graduates had to overcome was name recognition. Most of the patients in the new locations were unfamiliar with the term "osteopathy." To spread the word about their practices, most of the DOs advertised in the local newspapers. These advertisements explained that osteopathy was a new and effective method of treating disease that did not require the use of medication. Another form of advertisement included glowing testimonials by satisfied patients. Some advertisements consisted of attacks on MDs who, according to the ads, were poisoning their patients with drugs. One DO's advertisement went so far as to claim that local MDs were in cahoots with the local undertakers! (The DO landed in court and was forced to leave the area.[28]) Needless to say, this sort of advertisement angered the local MDs and assured their resistance to the profession. The most effective method of advertising was word of mouth. Patients who had experienced good results told others about the new DO in town.[29]

It had become evident early on that osteopathic medicine was more effective in treating chronic disease than in treating acute disease, and the usual course of treatment for chronic conditions often extended over a protracted period of time. The AOA considered this challenge on a national level and developed an official policy on treatment. Rather than charging by the visit, DOs would bill the patient on a monthly basis, usually $25. If treatment lasted longer than the month, a prorated charge was made. It was also recognized that more than three treatments a week exhausted both the patient and the doctor. Hence the policy was that the $25 fee covered three visits a week for a period of a month. Such price fixing would no doubt result in a prompt visit by a governmental agency or the Medical Board in today's environment.

At first, osteopaths were regarded as harmless quacks by the MDs, but as time passed it became evident that this "cult" was not going away. Opposition to the profession grew, with local MDs initiating actions to have DOs thrown in jail for practicing medicine without a license. Usually by the time a court appearance was set, the DO was supported by a large number of patients who had experienced successful treatments at the hands of the DO. As a result, these cases were usually thrown out of court. In Minnesota, Charles Still, DO, son of A. T. Still, was called upon to treat nearly seventy children who had diphtheria. The local MDs had had no success and had given up hope for saving the lives of these children. Using the osteopathic concepts and methods he had learned, Still was able to save all but one of the children. Local MDs encouraged the State Board of Health to arrest Still for practicing medicine without a license, but by the time the case came to court, there was such a public outcry that the MDs did not appear and the case was dropped.[30]

In several states, legislatures were called upon to develop laws that would allow the practice of osteopathy. The terms "medicine" or "medical practice" were considered the exclusive purview of MDs. State laws defined and limited osteopathy to the scope of practice taught by Still, including only osteopathic manipulation, obstetrics, and minor surgery. No major surgery or prescription of medication was permitted. These restrictions were soon modified in states with larger DO populations; however, in other states, such as Oregon, they continued for many years.

Endnotes

1. Norman Gevitz, *The DOs*, 8
2. Ibid., 10
3. Ibid., 9
4. Ibid., 10
5. Ibid.
6. Ibid., 11
7. Kay Atwood, *An Honorable History*, 4
8. Norman Gevitz, *The DOs*, 3
9. Ibid., 4
10. Ibid., 11
11. Ibid., 16; 8–15
12. Ibid., 17, 18
13. Ibid., 19
14. Lois Gant, ed., *One Hundred Years of Osteopathic Medicine,* 20; Gevitz, *The DOs*, 20
15. Norman Gevitz, *The DOs*, 20, 22
16. Ibid., 22
17. Ibid., 23
18. Ibid., 31
19. Lois Gant, ed., *One Hundred Years of Osteopathic Medicine,* 22
20. Norman Gevitz, *The DOs*, 26
21. Ibid., 48

22. Ibid., 39
23. Thomas A. Quinn, *The Feminine Touch,* 11
24. Ibid., 12
25. Norman Gevitz, *The DOs*, 52
26. Ibid., 39
27. Ibid., 37, 59
28. Ibid., 45
29. Ibid., 42–43
30. Ibid., 45

Section Two

Osteopathy Comes to Oregon

CHAPTER 2

Oregon in the Early Days

Until the Lewis and Clark expedition of 1804, the main interest in the Northwest was the fur trade. The British Hudson's Bay Company initially laid claim to the entire area through the trading posts they established along the major rivers that flowed to the Pacific. After President Jefferson gave the task of exploring the area to Lewis and Clark, the influx of emigrants began. Many traveled over the infamous Oregon Trail, an arduous trek made by pioneers traveling by ox-drawn wagons formed into "trains." Many died along the way, but those that made it were tough, self-sufficient people with a deep sense of purpose. As the fur trade played out, the British presence in the area diminished, but some, like John McLaughlin, a key leader of the Hudson's Bay Company, stayed and played important roles in the survival of the early settlers.[1]

The Donation Land Grant Act passed by Congress in 1850 offered incentive to settlers to move west. The law allowed a married man 320 acres and a single man 160 acres. Thousands of families from the Midwest and South came seeking a new beginning, and in 1859, just nine years after the Land Grant Act, Oregon became the thirty-third state.[2]

With the coming of the railroads, the demographics of the state changed very quickly. The population grew from a census estimate in 1870 of 81,000 to over 400,000 by 1900. People from all walks of life flocked to Oregon to start new lives. Because many of the new settlers were farmers, farms and farming communities sprang up, especially in the fertile Willamette Valley. The railroads made it possible to export crops to markets far away.[3]

But there were many other aspects to the Oregon economy. From the early 1850s until the 1860s, there was a thriving gold mining industry in southern and eastern Oregon. On the Oregon Coast, the salmon canning industry was booming; Astoria in particular benefited from the profits of that industry. With the widespread use of steam-powered logging machinery and saw mills, steadily increasing supplies of lumber, shingles, and other wood products were exported to markets around the world. By 1910, the timber industry had become the number one industry in the state.[4]

From 1848 to 1852, Oregon City, which marked the end of the Oregon Trail, was the capital of the Oregon Territory. The capital was moved to Salem in 1852, and continued as the state capital when Oregon became a state in 1859. About the same time, Portland supplanted Oregon City as the commercial hub of northern Oregon and the southern area of what would later become Washington State.[5]

Smaller towns sprang up to support industries in their areas. Towns such as Jacksonville and Medford to the south; Roseburg, Eugene, Albany, and Brownsville in the central area; and Salem further north came into being to provide homes, schools, churches, stores, and saloons for the workers and their families. Doctors usually located their offices in the larger of these towns, but often traveled by horse and buggy on a circuit that visited smaller towns, farms, and worksites in need of their services.

Travel was difficult. Dense, fast-growing underbrush and vast stands of timber made road building very challenging. Because of the rainy climate, the roads that did exist were a morass of mud for much of the year. Homesteaders and farmers usually had only primitive trails leading to their holdings, so access to these homesteads was challenging, and they were often not easy to find. A doctor attempting to respond to an emergency, such as a difficult home delivery, often arrived hours late. In some areas, such as the Willamette River Valley, travel between towns was possible by steamboat or later by rail.

The state was populated by a mixture of many races. The Native Americans had by this time been largely decimated by disease and were not a significant part of the population. The "establishment" consisted of the descendants of the employees of the Hudson's Bay Company, the survivors of the Oregon Trail treks, and their descendants. New emigrants from other nations, including a sizeable contingent of Scandinavians, began to arrive in large numbers. Because of their skills in logging, fishing, and lumber milling, many Swedes, Norwegians, and Finns were recruited by these industries. Other itinerant workers from around the world were welcomed to provide manpower for work in the forests and saw mills. (Often these were single men who only went by a first name; if they were killed in an accident, locating the next of kin was almost impossible.) Each ethnic group had it own customs, language, and methods for treating disease.

According to the United States Census at the time, the average life expectancy was estimated to be around fifty years of age.[6] There were regular epidemics of smallpox, yellow fever, malaria, tuberculosis, typhus, cholera, polio, scarlet fever, varicella, measles, chickenpox, bloody flux (gastroenteritis secondary to food poisoning), pneumonia, and influenza. The Native American population was especially hard hit and was nearly wiped out by these diseases. Childbirth-related and infant deaths were common. Childhood mortality was also very high, often from diseases that are today prevented by immunizations or treated by antibiotics.[7]

Aside from disease, there were many dangers associated with industry. Because great wealth was attainable from the natural resources abundant in Oregon, production was king. The timber and mining industries were particularly dangerous. There were no safety regulations. If a worker was injured on the job, it was usually considered the worker's own fault and it was his personal responsibility to get treatment. People died of wound infections on a regular basis. As the use of steam power grew, both the risk of injury to workers and the severity of the injuries increased.[8]

Physicians at the time struggled to do the best they could. Some were trained at medical schools, but most got their training as the apprentice of another doctor. Licensing was very permissive. Thanks to the Civil War, competence in treating trauma was usually satisfactory for the times, but tetanus and wound infections were still all too common. A few doctors performed certain types of surgeries, administrating ether via the drip method as anesthesia.

Medical treatment of disease at the time was chancy at best. Although the practice of bleeding was fading, there were still plenty of doctors who used this method. Other methods of treatment that had been in vogue for a long time were still widely used. The concept that disease was caused by something toxic in the colon or the stomach led to the use of powerful laxatives and emetics. Some of the more potent toxins known to man were used to treat disease. For example, strychnine was administered as a heart tonic, and drugs such as belladonna, antimony, digitalis (not standardized), tartar emetic, and lobelia were used. Calomel, a mercury compound used as a laxative, had a cumulative effect that produced brain damage and had other horrendous side effects.[9]

For the treatment of pain, many forms of opium and alcohol were widely available. Laudanum, a tincture containing both opium and alcohol, was a particularly popular. A popular formulation for women was Lydia Pinkham's tonic, which contained eighteen percent alcohol and is still available today. Cocaine was also widely available but somewhat more expensive. Unfortunately, addiction to these narcotic and alcoholic substances was quite common.

Most diseases were treated at home using remedies handed down through the generations. These remedies were readily available in local stores. Many ethnic groups had their own customs and methods for treating disease; for example, the Chinese workers imported to work in the mines and on the railroads brought with them the medicines that they had used in their native land. Ing Hay was a Chinese practitioner who used herbal remedies and Chinese methods of treatment with great success. He is memorialized in a small park in the town of John Day, Oregon.[10]

People feared the treatments prescribed by the local doctors and only resorted to their care when all else failed. But complex fractures, lacerations, and gunshot wounds were usually beyond the skills of the typical home health caregiver and were treated by the local doctors. Wound infections and tetanus were common complications. Childbirth usually occurred in the home with a family member or a neighbor in attendance, but if complications arose, a doctor or a midwife would be called to attend. There were few hospitals outside of Portland, so local doctors created "infirmaries" in their own homes or houses close by where they could perform surgeries and care for patients who required more intense treatment. During epidemics, quarantine was the only public health measure in common use, and it was rigorously enforced by the local law establishment.[11]

To those who lived on the East Coast and in the Midwest, Oregon was part of the "Wild West." Living conditions were primitive and expectations of quality medical care were low. This was the environment that existed when the first DOs entered Oregon with their new ideas for medical treatment.

Endnotes

1. Vera Martin Lynch, *Free Land for Free Men*, 53
2. William Robbins, *Landscapes of Promise*, 84
3. Ibid., 110–115
4. Ibid., 118–141
5. Vera Martin Lynch, *Free Land for Free Men*, 152
6. U.S. Census 1900
7. Kay Atwood, *An Honorable History*, 8

8. Ibid., 12
9. Norman Gevitz, *The DOs*, 7
10. Jodi Varon, "Ing Hay (Doc Hay)," *The Oregon Encyclopedia,* 1
11. Kay Atwood, *An Honorable History*, 18

CHAPTER 3

Enter Osteopathy

By 1898, there already were osteopaths, also known as doctors of osteopathy (DOs), practicing in the Oregon. According to the 1900 US census, Guy and Eva Hoisington were located in Pendleton, and F. E. and Hezzie Moore were located in Baker City. Robert B. Northrup, J. E. Anderson, Otis and Mabel Akins, Walter Allard Rogers, and Leroy and Lundy Byron Smith were practicing in Portland. Leroy and Lundy Smith opened the first osteopathic infirmary on the fourth floor of the Oregonian Building. By 1907, there were sixty-seven DOs practicing in Oregon, twenty-four of whom practiced in Portland.[1] The remaining forty-three DOs set up practices in many of the small towns that sprang up to support the timber, mining, or fishing industries. In other words, they went where they had the best chance of success.[2]

These pioneer DOs faced a host of challenges. They presented themselves as physicians trained in a method of treating disease that was quite different from that provided by the medical establishment. The challenge was to convince the public that this radically different approach to treating disease—no drugs, plenty of rest, proper diet, exercise, and osteopathic manipulation—really worked. Manipulation of the body to create optimum conditions for the body to heal itself was particularly controversial.

Another challenge was to find patients who were willing to try this novel new approach. To gain wider exposure, many DOs joined local churches, service clubs, and fraternal organizations, and even entered politics. Almost all advertised in the local newspapers, and some of the prominent DOs, such as the Andersons and the Akins, were often mentioned in the society pages of the local newspapers. These time-tested methods of promoting a practice are still valid and invaluable in establishing a practice in a small town.[3]

It was in the small towns that the profession thrived. Once people recognized that these new "docs" were competent, they were accepted. Concerns about where the doctor was trained were not as important as the results achieved. However, if there were already established medical doctors (MDs) in the area, the DOs usually had a much more difficult time being accepted. The MDs' scorn for the profession was widespread and could be quite damaging. Often DOs were derided as "quacks" or charlatans. The reality was that the DOs represented some serious competition to the MDs for patients.

By 1900, the telephone was already in wide use. DOs were initially listed in the classified section of the telephone directory as "osteopathists," then "osteopaths," then "osteopathic physicians and surgeons." The "physicians and surgeons" listing was designed to include both dual-degree DOs/MDs and DOs who were not MDs. As time went by, the listings tended to reflect the battle inside the profession as to what should constitute a well-trained DO. Some years the only listing to be found was "osteopaths" with no separate listing for the dual-degree DOs; the dual-degree DOs were now listed under the MD listings.[4]

As the number of DOs increased across the country, the American Osteopathic Association (AOA) was formed in 1901. This organization soon developed subcommittees to address the many challenges facing the new profession. One committee was tasked with assisting the states in forming local organizations to further the cause of osteopathy, and to develop "model laws" to be adopted by states to regulate the osteopathic profession.[5]

The Oregon Osteopathic Association (OOA), later known as the

Osteopathic Physicians and Surgeons of Oregon (OPSO), was also formed in 1901. By 1906, the OOA had become an important voice in the state legislature as new laws were created to strengthen the Oregon Board of Medical Examiners and to add specific language regulating the osteopathic profession. The association officers included the names of several prominent and influential DOs: J. E. Anderson, President; Otis Akin, First Vice President; W. O. Flack, Second Vice President; Mabel Akin, Secretary; and F. J. Barr, Treasurer. (Anderson was based in Dallas, Oregon; all of the other officers were from Portland.) The association trustees were R. B. Northrup, G. I. Gates, and Mary T. Schoettle, all of Portland; W. L. Mercer of Salem; and Cynthia Ramsay of Albany.[6]

By 1907, the Oregon State Legislature had enacted regulations regarding the practices of osteopathic physicians. The Board of Medical Examiners was given the responsibility of examining and licensing all physicians in the state.

The licensing laws for DOs stated:

> Any person holding a diploma from an established school of osteopathy, recognized as of good standing and wherein the course of study comprises a term of at least 20 months, or (4) terms of (5) months each in actual attendance at such school, and which shall include instruction in the following branches, to wit: Anatomy, Physiology, Chemistry, Histology, Pathology, Gynecology, Obstetrics, theory of osteopathy, and two full terms of practice of osteopathy shall upon application and presentation of such diploma to the state board of medical examiners and satisfying such board that he is the legal holder thereof, be granted by such board an examination in said branches. The license provided for in the foregoing section shall not authorize the holder to prescribe or use drugs in his practice or perform major or operative surgery.[7]

Frederick Everett Moore, DO, was appointed by Governor Oswald West as the first DO member of the Board of Medical Examiners. He was the first DO whose signature appeared on Oregon medical licenses, beginning with those issued in 1908.

After this new law was enacted, there was a question as to whether the DOs already practicing in the state should be required to take the newly mandated examination. Since these doctors were already in practice, the Oregon attorney general's opinion was they should not be required to take the examination. Hence in January of 1908, all sixty-seven currently practicing DOs were given their new licenses on the same day.[8]

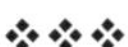

The typical osteopathic office consisted of a reception area with a desk where the doctor's secretary (often his spouse) sat to schedule appointments, collect fees (there was no insurance at the time), and chaperone the doctor when female exams were required. The office would also have a filing cabinet where the medical records, kept on 4x8 filing cards, were stored. On each card, the doctor would write a one-line report with the diagnosis, treatment, and fee. Behind the office was the treatment area. This usually was a single room with a treatment table, a light source, instrument cabinets, and the doctor's desk. In rural areas, there was often a second room devoted to obstetrics and surgery, and a small room for storing medications dispensed by the doctor. It was not unusual to find some sort of X-ray equipment as well. Patients undergoing minor surgeries were usually seen only once or twice, while patients who were being treated with osteopathic methods were usually seen at least three times a week. The patient was expected to pay cash at the time of the visit or make arrangements to pay on a monthly basis.[9]

In smaller towns, it was not unusual for the clinic to be in the doctor's home with the family residence upstairs or to the rear of the clinic. The doctor was expected to be on call twenty-four hours a day, seven days a week. Patients also expected the doctor to travel to them, not vice versa. Traveling to outlying areas on unpaved and often muddy roads was difficult and time-consuming. The automobile eventually supplanted the horse and buggy, but the barriers of mud and poor quality roads did not improve until much later.

Some DOs elected to practice in larger towns and cities where the roads were paved and public transportation was available. Despite these improvements, the practice of house calls continued, and it was an established routine for many osteopathic primary care doctors. In the home setting, the doctor could learn important information about his patient's situation that would never have been apparent in the office setting. Administering osteopathic manipulative therapy could be challenging in a home setting, but with a sound knowledge of biomechanics and a lot of ingenuity, DOs were able to incorporate these therapies during a house call.

In Portland and some of the larger towns, DOs located their practices in the larger, more modern buildings located downtown, often in the same buildings as dentists and MDs. Even though they were located in the same buildings, it was considered unethical for MDs to accept referrals from DOs.[10] This policy reflected the political power of the American Medical Association (AMA) and the Oregon Medical Association (OMA). However, if patient welfare was threatened, this policy was not enforced.

When a DO needed to refer a patient to a specialist, problems could arise. If a DO general practitioner (GP) referred a patient to an MD specialist, the MD would often make disparaging remarks about the DO and urge that patient to seek the services of a local MD. When this occurred, DOs would spread the word about these hostile MDs, and DOs would no longer refer to them. To overcome problems with hostile MD specialists, DO GPs who had a special interest or showed expertise in a particular area of medicine (dermatology or gynecology, for example) would consult on patients referred to them by fellow DOs. The DO specialists would then refer the patients back to their original DO GP.

Hospitalization situations could also cause problems. At the time, DOs did not have hospital privileges, so a DO patient taken to a local hospital for emergency treatment would be assigned a local MD at the hospital. This MD would continue care after the patient was discharged from the hospital, and the DO who had been the patient's doctor would never be notified. Hospitalization issues could sometimes be overcome by dual-degree DOs who could arrange for major surgical care in the local hospitals that were off limits to regular DOs.

Although most childbirth deliveries continued to be in the home setting, affluent expectant mothers in larger towns would be admitted to a hospital or infirmary to have their babies. The mother and infant remained in the hospital or infirmary for another seven to ten days after the delivery. Then the mother and baby were transferred home by ambulance, where the mother would have another seven to ten days of rest before she resumed her normal routine. One woman, whose husband was an osteopathic medical student at the Des Moines Osteopathic Medical School, delivered at the osteopathic hospital in Des Moines, Iowa. Her husband was moonlighting at a local funeral home at the time, and drove his wife and new baby home in a hearse. She was on a stretcher in the back, waving happily to passersby—a strange sight to those who noticed.[11]

By 1910, the number of DOs starting new practices in Oregon had diminished.[12] The laws governing the practice of osteopathic medicine were quite specific, and young doctors who were now receiving more education in medical school found it increasingly difficult to limit themselves to the model of practice laid down by A. T. Still. However, the established DOs were enjoying great success using Still's classic training. Why rock the boat?

This attitude created a conflict between those DOs who advocated for the continued application of the methods espoused by Still and those who were incorporating more modern treatments. Over time, this conflict had profound effects on the history of the osteopathic profession.

Endnotes

1. Oregon Medical Board and City of Portland telephone directories
2. 1900 Census; The Oregonian, Feb. 1, 1900; City of Portland telephone directories
3. 1910 Census
4. City of Portland telephone directories, 1900–1925
5. Norman Gevitz, *The DOs*, 54
6. Journal of American Osteopathic Association, 1906
7. Lord's Oregon Laws, 1907
8. List furnished to the author by the Oregon Medical Association
9. Norman Gevitz, *The DOs*, 63
10. Ibid., 157
11. See J. Scott Heatherington biography (page 120)
12. Membership in the OOA leveled off after the new rules were written and the number of DOs remained about the same until the 1960s.

CHAPTER 4

Expanding the Scope of Practice

With the exception of dual-degree DOs, the first doctors of osteopathic medicine practicing in Oregon were trained by and used the methods originally taught by A. T. Still. Prior to 1907, all medical practitioners were allowed to practice using the methods taught in their respective medical schools, but after 1907, all medical professions were licensed and supervised by the Oregon Board of Medical Examiners.[1]

Many practicing MDs at the time were the products of medical schools, homeopathic schools, or eclectic schools that were of marginal quality, or they had completed an apprenticeship with a recognized MD. The key to medical practice was a diploma from a medical school or an apprenticeship, and the ability to pass a basic examination of medical knowledge administered by the Board of Medical Examiners.[2]

Osteopathic medicine was little understood at the time. In an attempt to better regulate the practices of the DOs in the state, the Board of Medical Examiners went to the Oregon legislature and asked for more formal rules. These new regulations were enacted in 1907, and for the first time, DOs were officially prohibited from prescribing medication or performing major surgeries in Oregon.[3] It was at this time that a DO became a formal member of the Board of Medical Examiners to represent the interests of osteopathic physicians in Oregon.

When the new rules went into effect in 1908, there were sixty-seven DOs practicing in Oregon. A few were dual-degree DOs, and these were permitted by their MD degrees to continue to perform major surgeries and prescribe medication.

The majority of the DOs practiced using the principles espoused by Still: normalizing vascular, lymphatic, and musculoskeletal function through manipulation, and advocating for a healthier lifestyle and the avoidance of medications, tobacco, and alcohol. These osteopathic physicians were called ten-finger, traditional, or classic DOs; the dual-degree DOs who could prescribe medication were called three-finger DOs (the number of fingers needed to hold a pen to write a prescription).

By 1908, there were already important advances in medicine in general. Vaccines, public health measures, and other important discoveries began to change how medicine was practiced.[4] DOs trained in the early years enjoyed success with the traditional methods, but later osteopathic medical school graduates and others were anxious to use these medical advances in the treatment of their patients. In the AOA and nationally, the trend for greater acceptance of medical advances and their incorporation into osteopathic education and practice was gaining momentum. The traditionalists were gradually giving way to the more progressive DOs.[5]

Then the great flu epidemic of 1916–19 struck, taking an estimated 668,000 lives in the United States alone, many of them young adults.[6] This was a time when osteopathic methods were put to the test. DOs around the country were reporting success in treating flu patients with osteopathic methods that mobilized the spine and the lymphatics of the respiratory system (e.g., Thoracic Pump Method).

At the time of the epidemic, the AOA was still trying to convince the War Department that DOs should be allowed to be military doctors. The president of the AOA put out a call to all DOs requesting that they report their results in the treatment of influenza. Their results were submitted to the *Journal of the Osteopathic Association* and *The Osteopathic Physician*. Between October 1918 and June 1919, a total of 2,445 DOs submitted their results to these journals. Of the 11,120 influenza cases treated by DOs during this time period, there were only 257 deaths or 0.2 percent from all influenza cases treated. Of the 6,258 pneumonia cases treated by DOs, there were only 635 fatalities or 10.1 percent of all cases.[7] These results were compared to a ten to fifteen percent death rate from influenza and a twenty-five percent death rate from pneumonia reported by doctors using methods advocated by William Osler and other leading MDs.[8]

Both nationally and in Oregon, traditionalist DOs used these successes to thwart further moves to incorporate the advances in medicine. Progress in convincing legislatures to write new statutes broadening the scope of practice for DOs was lost. Osteopathic schools that had begun to teach materia medica and pharmacology were forced to abandon those portions of their curricula. In 1917, the AOA Board of Trustees adopted a position paper called *The Profession's Policy* that instructed osteopathic schools to teach only osteopathic principles, with no instruction in materia medica or pharmacology. State legislatures were encouraged to use these policies as a regulatory template for laws applying to the osteopathic profession. At the urging of Oregon DOs, the state legislature went further and adopted a regulation forbidding the Oregon Board of Medical Examiners from even accepting an application for licensure from a DO who had graduated from an osteopathic medical school where materia medica or pharmacology was taught.[9]

As long as the AOA maintained tight control of the curricula of the osteopathic schools, newly minted DOs were not trained in a formal way in materia medica and pharmacology. A mounting pressure to change these policies came from students and doctors across the country. In 1924, at the request of its students and alumni, the Chicago College of Osteopathic Medicine tried to expand the curriculum offered by the college to include instruction in materia medica and pharmacology. When the school approached the AOA

Board for permission to add these topics to their curriculum, the Board refused and advised the school administrators that if they proceeded the school would lose its accreditation.

Pressure on the AOA continued, and the older, more traditional Board members were replaced. Finally, in 1927, policies limiting materia medica and pharmacology began to change. At first, classes termed "comparative therapeutics" were cautiously added to the school catalogs; by 1929, materia medica and pharmacology were being offered by all of the osteopathic medical schools.

At this point, the law codes regulating the profession in Oregon adhered strictly to AOA policies. In states with larger DO populations (Michigan, Ohio, Pennsylvania, Missouri, Iowa, Texas, and California), the state legislatures were more willing to adopt these curriculum changes. In Oregon, however, change came very slowly, and it wasn't until the 1920s that DOs with training in materia medica and pharmacology were permitted to apply for licensure. In 1927, the rules prohibiting DOs from prescribing medication or performing major surgery were finally changed.[10]

By the 1930s, the character of the membership of the AOA House of Delegates and the Board of Directors began to change. Many of the traditionalist members who had been trained by Still or at the osteopathic medical schools that adhered to a strict traditional curriculum had retired. These doctors were replaced by physicians who recognized that medicine had changed dramatically and that the osteopathic concept of disease being attributed to spinal misalignment and treatable with manipulation to free the body's natural ability to heal itself was incomplete. The discoveries and treatments of modern medicine could no longer be denied. The goal of these doctors was not to discard manipulation, but to consider manipulation techniques as tools to be used along with the discoveries and treatments of modern medicine, thereby creating more well-rounded physicians who were able to offer more treatment options to their patients.[11]

To meet the increasing demands of the state licensure boards and the students themselves, schools of osteopathic medicine began to institute important changes:

- Premedical educational requirements were increased to a minimum of high school graduation and at least two years of college.
- The standard duration of education was increased to a three-year curriculum for a time, then to the four-year curriculum used to this day.
- PhDs were brought in to teach basic sciences.
- The physical plants of the schools were enlarged and enhanced to allow for more and better-equipped laboratories.
- Hospitals were constructed or enlarged at each of the medical schools, allowing more education at the hospital level.[12]

These changes were costly to the schools. Tuition had to be drastically increased, and many applicants were unable to qualify under the increased admission standards. Many osteopathic institutions were legitimately concerned whether they could survive at all. Yet despite these challenges and in the midst of the greatest economic crisis the country had ever experienced, the osteopathic medical schools survived. This is a testimony to the strong support of the osteopathic profession at large.[13]

By the late 1930s, most states were also requiring a one-year rotating internship for licensure. Initially, DOs were scoring very poorly on state licensure exams, barely above chiropractors. The premedical requirements and duration of education for DOs and chiropractors were similar. (Daniel David Palmer, founder of what he termed chiropractic, was in fact an early student of A. T. Still who disagreed with Still's approach and founded his own school in Davenport, Iowa.[14]) The difference was that osteopathic colleges emphasized the skills that one would require from an osteopathic general practice physician, while chiropractic training focused primarily on manipulation.

With the push by state medical legislatures for an improved and more extensive education for DOs, state licensing examination test scores by DOs began to improve dramatically and soon were comparable to their MD counterparts. Oregon legislators noticed these results and enacted new statutes that allowed DOs to perform major surgery and write prescriptions.

In some states, reciprocity of licensure from one state to another was allowed, but in Oregon, candidates for licensure continued to be examined locally. This examination covered general medicine, surgery, public health, and obstetrics. It also covered topics pertaining to the laws governing the practice of medicine in Oregon.

Despite the difficult economic times of the late 1920s and 1930s, people still required care. DOs found that their unique ability to provide osteopathic manipulative care along with traditional medical care assured a steady stream of patients coming to their offices. In fact, a review of the classified sections of the City of Portland telephone directory reveals that the population of DOs practicing in the community showed little change in numbers from the 1900s, even during the Great Depression.

Despite the changes in the laws regulating the practice of osteopathic medicine in Oregon, most DOs were rather slow to adopt the medical advances of the time, including prescribing medication or performing major surgery. Prescriptions written by DOs were challenged by pharmacists, nurses, and county medical societies; based on these complaints, DOs were charged by the Board of Medical Examiners for practicing medicine without a license. The primary treatment methods by most DOs continued to be based on osteopathic principles.

There was another interesting challenge presented by this broader scope of practice. Most patients who came to DOs were accustomed to being treated exclusively with osteopathic methods and came to the DOs for that express reason. The general public was slow to accept a DO who could prescribe medication and perform general surgery.

From the mid-1930s onward, graduates of the osteopathic medical schools that offered the expanded curriculum, such as the California College of Osteopathic Medicine in Los Angeles, were well qualified to practice in urban and rural areas. Yet recognition by the medical community was far in the future. While state legislatures recognized the expanded education and capabilities of DOs, MDs increased their resistance on a community level and the profession was now officially labeled as a cult.[15] DOs continued to be branded as "quacks" who really didn't know what they were doing. Throughout the country, DOs continued to be barred from practicing in public or charitable hospitals.

Endnotes

1. Lord's Oregon Laws 1907
2. Ibid.
3. Ibid.
4. Norman Gevitz, *The DOs*, 73
5. Ibid., 84
6. Ibid., 82
7. Ibid.
8. Ibid., 81–82
9. Ibid., 80
10. Ibid., 84
11. Ibid., 94
12. Ibid., 94–98
13. Ibid., 94–100
14. Ibid., 66–68
15. Official Policy of the American Medical Society and followed by the Oregon Medical Society.

Section Three

Overcoming Obstacles

CHAPTER 5

Osteopathic Infirmaries and Hospitals

Osteopathic infirmaries and hospitals were first created to accommodate the often lengthy nature of osteopathic treatment. However, these facilities later became necessary because DOs were restricted from practicing in most public hospitals, first under law and later due to the policies of the AMA.

The First Infirmaries and Hospitals

After A. T. Still became established in Kirksville, Missouri, people from all over the country came for treatment by the doctor, and later by the doctor and his students at the American School of Osteopathy. Usually these patients required more than one treatment session to achieve the results they were seeking, so hotels sprang up to accommodate these patients. Patients requiring more intensive treatment were treated at an infirmary attached to the clinics and the school.

In 1906, the American School of Osteopathic Medicine Hospital was formed and afforded students training and experience in surgery and obstetrics as well as in the care of the very ill.[1] A few months later, a school of nursing was formed in affiliation with the hospital. The students received instruction in the latest nursing methods and specialized education in osteopathic medicine. The original hospital became so busy that a second hospital, the Laughlin Osteopathic Hospital, was opened just across the street. Both hospitals offered nursing programs that were very well received. Between 1906 and 1918, two more specialty hospitals were added. The first was devoted to ophthalmology and refraction, and offered fourth-year osteopathic medical students specialized training in dealing with the eye. The other facility, called the Missouri Woman's Hospital, specialized in obstetrics and gynecological services in a hospital setting.[2]

In 1925, the American School of Osteopathy (ASO), the original school founded by A. T. Still in 1892, merged with the A. T. Still College of Osteopathic Medicine (founded in 1922 by George and Blanche Laughlin and located just two blocks away from the original school) to form the A. T. Still University College of Osteopathic Medicine. George Still, DO, son of A. T. Still, was president of ASO until he was killed in a tragic hunting accident in 1922 and the surviving board was unable to provide the leadership required to maintain the school. The two nursing schools also merged and were highly successful until they were closed in 1949.[3]

Infirmaries and Hospitals in Oregon

Outside of Missouri and a few other states (Michigan, Ohio, California, and Pennsylvania), DOs were not accorded the same reception and privileges that they were accustomed to while in training. In Oregon, the laws enacted in 1907 clearly stated that DOs were required to limit their practice to osteopathic medicine as taught by Still, and, while they were trained in manipulation, surgery, and obstetrics, they were not permitted to prescribe medication or to perform major surgery.

Most vexing was the fact that DOs were totally prohibited from gaining privileges or practicing in state-supported or charitable hospitals across the country. To care for their more seriously ill patients, Oregon DOs had to rely on home health care provided by the families of the patient. The doctor would make daily house calls to attend to these patients.

To attend to patients that required care but lived too far to make house calls practicable, doctors would purchase a residence and convert it into an infirmary where trained staff, sometimes an RN, would be in attendance. On occasion, a doctor would perform a surgery and then transfer the patient to the infirmary for recovery, releasing them when they could safely be cared for at home. At the time, it was customary after delivery that a mother and her baby would be kept at rest before they were deemed ready to go home. Infirmaries were very useful for this type of care as well. When an infirmary was not readily available, a doctor might rent a room at a local hotel and hire a medical person, such as an RN, to tend these patients while they were under observation. In The Dalles, Floyd Logue, DO, used this method to care for ailing patients who resided too far from town for daily visits.

In smaller towns, MDs would create privately owned proprietary hospitals where patient volume trumped AMA and OMA rules, thus allowing busy DOs to care for their patients in a hospital setting.

In the larger Oregon cities—such as Portland, Salem, and Eugene—access to hospitals by DOs was strictly banned. This led to the creation of osteopathic infirmaries like the one created in 1900 by C. T. and L. B. Smith in the old Oregonian Building in Portland, which became an osteopathic sanitarium in 1907. In the 1930s, a cancer center was opened in Portland, and in 1940, the first osteopathic hospital was formed by O. F. Heisley on NE 20th Street in Portland. Attached to that hospital was the Mar-Dur Hospital, which specialized in emergency care.[4] DOs who were well trained in surgery and pharmacology manned these facilities.

Even when the practice rights of DOs were no longer restricted by law, DOs were still blocked from practicing in most Oregon hospitals, due to the policies of the AMA and the OMA. When patients required major surgery or treatments not available in the infirmaries, local DOs turned to dual-degree colleagues who had obtained MD degrees.

During WWII, many MDs were drafted into the armed forces, but DOs were banned from the military. As a result, more DOs began to locate to areas where there were few doctors; indeed, the DO might be the only doctor in the area. In a few towns, such as Ontario, Oregon, the ban on DOs practicing in MD hospitals was ignored for the duration of WWII. For example, at Holy Rosary Hospital in Ontario, Larry Jones, DO, served the community by handling the hospital emergency room and delivering a multitude of babies. But after the war, he was again banned from the hospital and even from the weekly continuing medical education (CME) sessions held at the hospital.

Some Oregon towns were not as accommodating. Dr. George Larson II set up practice in Brownsville, Oregon, and served that community as almost the only doctor. Larson was expected to be on call twenty-four hours a day, seven days a week. He often tended injured loggers and mill workers onsite. If hospitalization was required, he had to bypass the MD hospital in Lebanon and bring his patients to the osteopathic hospital in Albany, a much longer drive. To assure as speedy a trip as possible, the city fathers of Brownsville fitted Larson's car with a siren because he personally transported many of his patients to the hospital in Albany.

While the official position of the AMA and OMA on DOs practicing in MD-dominated hospitals remained unchanged, the attitude of the patients was much different. Many of the patients who had been cared for by DOs in their communities remained loyal and were strong supporters of the profession in the state legislature and in the movement to form freestanding osteopathic hospitals where osteopathic medical services could be provided.

In 1944, a group of DOs and local businessmen in Portland purchased a nursing home and converted it into a hospital. It was not a convenient facility—patients often had to be carried upstairs for surgery or delivery—but it was a bona fide hospital.[5]

In 1945, the first intern class (Doctors Barr and Wessen) graduated from the Portland Osteopathic Hospital. The hospital's initial facility was located on 616 NW 18th Street. Although the structure was old and inconvenient, it became a nexus of osteopathic practice in the area. A staff of osteopathic specialist physicians—including surgeons, anesthesiologists, radiologists, an EENT specialist, and an internist—worked at the facility regularly. Major surgeries were performed, babies were delivered, and use of the hospital by the GPs in the area assured operation at full capacity.[6] About the same time Portland Osteopathic Hospital was created, other small osteopathic hospitals were opened around the state.

Later, with financial assistance from hospital staff and from Hill Burton Funds (money from the federal government to finance the construction of hospitals), a new Portland Osteopathic Hospital was built in the Eastmoreland area on Steele Street close to the campus of Reed College. When the facility was moved, it was renamed Eastmoreland General Hospital.[7]

When Portland Osteopathic relocated to the Eastmoreland location, a group of DOs created their own hospital in Forest Grove, Oregon. At almost the same time, the following osteopathic hospitals were also established: Eugene Osteopathic Hospital, Dallas Osteopathic Hospital, Albany Osteopathic Hospital, Crater General Hospital in Medford, and Canyonville Hospital in Myrtle Creek.

Each hospital was formed and staffed by a small group of DOs. Of necessity, each member was required to wear several hats: chief of staff, medical director, medical education director, chief of surgery, chief of obstetrics, and so on. These hospitals offered basic services such as surgery, X-rays, obstetrics, and laboratory services. The emergency room (often quite busy) was manned on a rotating basis by all of the doctors on the staff. All of these hospitals had at least one AOA board-certified general surgeon who was required to handle any sort of surgery that came in the door. A DO radiologist, who was either "in house" or provided service on a rotating basis, provided X-ray services. Anesthesia was assigned to a staff member who was familiar with the "ether drip" method of anesthesia. Often the hospital had one general internist on staff who would serve as a consultant and manage the more complex cases. The GPs on staff usually managed their own cases but would consult with the internist when needed. For other specialties, DO consultants would travel from Portland to DO hospitals in other communities on a regular schedule. Despite the official discouragement of the practice by the OMA and AMA, certain MD specialists would also act as consultants on difficult cases.[8]

Robert Butler, DO, one of the anesthesiologists at Portland Osteopathic Hospital, ran a training program for DO anesthesiologists from other parts of the state. At the time, several of the "anesthesiologists" were GPs who had been chosen to administer ether drip anesthesia at their hospitals. Butler trained these doctors in airway management and the use of more modern anesthetics.[9]

Specialists would rent an office close to the hospital where they could consult on patients. Occasionally an MD consultant or surgeon would visit as well. Only Portland Osteopathic Hospital (later Eastmoreland Hospital) offered internships and a residency training program in family practice. But the other DO hospitals usually welcomed students or residents who wished to be mentored by a staff member.

Compared to the MD facilities in the same communities, these hospitals were tiny, usually operating on a very tight budget. Even in their heyday they were often near financial insolvency. Hospital success depended on the loyal support of the osteopathic physicians who were on staff, so one of the most challenging tasks faced by hospital administrators was keeping these admitting doctors happy.

The RNs and other hospital personnel were often people who had benefited from osteopathic treatment. They were committed to assuring the success of the profession in the hospital arena. The nurses especially played an important role in the training of students and interns. They often had key roles in the decision-making processes affecting the everyday care of the patients. The small size of these hospitals assured the patients of excellent personalized care that was never possible in the large MD-dominated facilities, thus garnering the loyal support of the patients. Sadly, the preferences of patients were often trumped by insurance plans that had exclusive contracts with the large hospitals.

Hospital boards were often made up in part by business people and others who had benefited from osteopathic care. Another group that was instrumental in the success of the hospital was the auxiliary. These spouses and other women worked tirelessly to raise money to decorate the hospital, provide scholarships to students, work in the gift shops, and provide other support services. These women and volunteers from the community were indeed an important part of the hospital.

By the 1960s, the national outright prohibition on DOs being on the staff of MD hospitals began to be lifted. Primary care DOs were wooed into joining MD hospitals which were geographically much closer to where their offices were located. For instance, instead of a forty-mile trip to and from Eastmoreland Hospital, Dr. Ned Davies of Canby could travel twelve miles to the Oregon City Hospital, a major convenience for him and his patients. In this case, the small town location of so many DOs actually worked against them. They sincerely wanted to continue to support the osteopathic hospital, but referring to Eastmoreland Hospital was much less convenient than the local MD hospital. Initially, these DOs were not permitted to manage their patients in the MD hospital setting, but they could "visit" their patients there.[10]

The Vietnam War finally caused the last barriers to both military service and general practice to fall. It soon became evident that the old policy of banning DO physicians from military service was depriving the military of a pool of well-trained primary care physicians, so this policy was changed. Once allowed to serve, DOs distinguished themselves in the military, and with the policy of merit-based promotion, many were promoted to important positions. If they could do a good job in the military, they certainly should be allowed to receive full practice rights in the local MD hospitals.[11]

One of the last barriers to fall was the acceptance of osteopathically trained interns to MD specialty training programs. This final barrier to DO specialists was lifted thanks to the efforts of Rolland

O'Dell, DO, board certified cardiologist, and others. Today, one can find DO specialists in virtually every hospital in Oregon.

In the 1970s, osteopathic hospitals across the nation began to face serious challenges to their continued economic survival. When MD-dominated hospitals were opened to DOs, the DOs found it more convenient, for both their patients and for them, to use the MD hospitals, which were usually much closer than an osteopathic hospital. Admissions, length of stay, and medical necessity issues also contributed to the decrease in reimbursements to osteopathic hospitals. Many of these hospitals also had internship and residency programs that were financial obligations. Unlike their MD-dominated counterparts, osteopathic hospitals could not rely on endowments and charitable giving to sustain them. Even though a group of extremely loyal DOs continued to admit to and support these hospitals, this was not enough, and economic pressures forced many of the small osteopathic hospitals across the country to close their doors. In Oregon, the small osteopathic hospitals were either acquired by larger institutions or closed. Eastmoreland Hospital was the last surviving osteopathic hospital in Oregon.[12]

Recognizing that hospital admissions were decreasing, grants to doctors who wished to enlarge their practices and other inducements were tried, all to no avail. When doctors tried to admit patients to an osteopathic hospital, they were frustrated by the rules of health maintenance organizations (HMOs) and other roadblocks. Eastmoreland Hospital was not an HMO-approved facility, which meant that the patients would have to cover the added expense of being cared for in an "out of plan" hospital. Medicare patients not restricted by some HMOs or other medical plans could be admitted, but reimbursements were often far less than the actual cost of caring for the patient. Patients enrolled in FamilyCare (an HMO for Medicaid patients) could be admitted, but the Medicaid reimbursements were also quite low. By law, the hospital was required to maintain an emergency room, and, as has been the experience of other hospitals with emergency rooms, up to forty-five percent of patients had no insurance and no means to pay. Somehow the hospital was able to sustain the salaries of the residents who called Eastmoreland Hospital their base.

In 1984, the Board of Directors and the medical staff of Eastmoreland Hospital determined that the only way for the hospital to continue operation was to merge with another hospital group. After considerable negotiation, the hospital was purchased for $4.5 million by American Hospital Management (AHM), a national firm. Later, Eastmoreland was bundled with Woodland Park Hospital and both entities were managed by AHM; however, in time it became evident that these two hospitals were unprofitable and were sold to another hospital corporation. A succession of owners ensued until the last owner abruptly closed Eastmoreland Hospital and auctioned off all the equipment in 2004. The structure was razed by Reed College, the new owners. A few privately owned bricks remain to remind the DO community of this once vibrant little hospital.

The closure of Eastmoreland Hospital came as a shock to the osteopathic physicians practicing in the greater Portland area. To many, it was their home, their "clubhouse," a place to meet to discuss cases with colleagues. Based on its past struggles, however, it was little short of miraculous that the hospital survived as long as it did.

Although Eastmoreland Hospital no longer exists, its legacy lives on. From 1945 (as Portland Osteopathic Hospital) until closure, 282 interns and residents graduated from Eastmoreland General Hospital; from 1988 until closure, seventy-three interns and residents received their training in the specialty of family practice. Many of these doctors are still in practice in Oregon.[13]

In addition, the proceeds from the sale of the hospital to AHM were used to form a nonprofit organization called the Northwest Osteopathic Medical Foundation with J. Scott Heatherington, DO, as the first president and David Rianda as the executive secretary. The mission of the Foundation has been the furtherance of the profession throughout the Northwest. To accomplish this mission, the Foundation has made donations to other charitable organizations in Oregon, offered scholarships to osteopathic medical students, put on child safety oriented programs such as "Kid Safe," and sponsored a medical information series for local television. The Foundation has also provided seed monies to fledgling osteopathic organizations in Idaho, Montana, and Alaska. When a new osteopathic medical school was being formed in Yakima, Washington, the Foundation pledged a $250,000 guaranty. Today, thanks to the financial skill of the lay members and doctors, the Foundation continues to be an important source of financial support to osteopathic students in the Northwest.

Endnotes

1. Thomas A. Quinn, *The Feminine Touch,* 54
2. Ibid., 59
3. Ibid., 161
4. City of Portland telephone directory 1930
5. See Neher biography (page 151)
6. See biographies of Neher (page 151), Henry (page 129), Butler (page 108), and Graham (page 117)
7. See biographies of Butler (page 108) and Browning (page 107)
8. See biographies of Bauers (page 99), Davies (page 114), and Carlstrom (page 111)
9. See Butler biography (page 108)
10. See Davies biography (page 114)
11. Norman Gevitz, *The DOs,* 143
12. See O'Dell biography (page 154)
13. Computer records rescued from Eastmoreland General Hospital by Beth Shelton, secretary to the hospital administrator

CHAPTER 6

Osteopathic Specialization

The development of osteopathic hospitals was important for another reason: they provided openings for various osteopathic specialists to set up practice in the state and provided facilities for training, internships, and residencies in specialty areas.

When osteopathy was in its infancy, the original goal of osteopathic education was to provide graduates with training in all of the areas of medicine that were commonly encountered in everyday practice. The need for specialization was a natural outgrowth of the rapidly increasing developments in medical knowledge.

As mentioned earlier, in the early days, DOs entering practice in Oregon and many other states found they were restricted by license to performing minor surgery and some obstetrics, but could not perform major surgery or prescribe medication. As a result, DOs restricted their practices to attending minor wounds, some fractures, and obstetrics. In 1917, a nationwide survey of DOs revealed that out of the fifty-two percent of DOs who were accepting obstetrics cases, the average practitioner handled less than five deliveries a year.[1] Most of the DOs across the country and especially in Oregon specialized in osteopathic manipulation.[2]

DOs who wished to perform major surgery or to practice in an MD-dominated hospital returned to medical school and obtained MD degrees. These dual-degree DOs played an important role in the osteopathic community, because primary care DOs could refer to a fellow DO rather than to an MD. DO GPs also developed areas of special interest and accepted referrals from their colleagues. For example, Mary Howells, DO (Kirksville 1911), devoted her career to psychiatry. Later, Frank Trostel, DO, became expert in the treatment of dermatological disorders; John Wood, DO, was a GP specializing in obstetrics; and Sheridan Thiringer, DO, specialized in anesthesiology.[3]

The Development of Osteopathic Specialties and Boards

General surgery was the first specialty to become recognized as the key to the operation of any hospital, MD or DO. The surgical residency as it is known today was unavailable in most osteopathic institutions. Most training in surgery was accomplished through apprenticeships and preceptorships.[4]

At the time, the scope of practice for surgery included the abdomen and all its contents. This included gynecological surgery, which comprised a large percentage of the cases performed by general surgeons, who considered gynecological organs an important part of their domain. By necessity, they also performed orthopedic surgery, and ear, nose, and throat procedures, such as thyroid and tonsil procedures. One surgeon even performed emergency dental procedures; according to the story, the result was less than stellar.[5]

Most surgeon apprentices or assistants served until they were deemed qualified to perform procedures on their own. Surgeons often supplemented their training by visiting outstanding teaching centers in the United States and Europe.

Usually, general surgeons played a dominant role in the administration of a hospital, often serving as CEOs and board chairmen. These surgeon CEOs had their own society, the American Hospital Administrators (osteopathic) (AHA). In 1927, this society was incorporated into the larger American College of Surgery (ACOS). In addition to hospital inspections, the ACOS made recommendations to the AOA regarding the qualifications for surgeons to operate in approved hospitals. Until the ACOS developed these standards, the only qualifications required to do surgery were those of the individual hospitals.

States such as California, Michigan, Ohio, Pennsylvania, Missouri, Arizona, Texas, New Jersey, and New York had both favorable licensing legislation and large concentrations of osteopathic physicians. These factors fostered the growth of osteopathic hospitals associated with the osteopathic medical schools as well as free-standing osteopathic hospitals. Surgeons at these osteopathic hospitals performed and taught major surgeries.

In earlier years, the ACOS had established a junior membership for young surgeons who were not yet qualified for senior membership. Prior to 1935, junior surgeons had to submit ten surgical cases and a scientific thesis. They also had to serve a one-year rotating internship in a satisfactory training facility or document that they had served a preceptorship under a surgeon with recognized qualifications. Surgeons who applied for senior membership were required to meet all the requirements for junior membership and to present twenty-five surgical case records acceptable to the ACOS Executive Committee. In addition, senior member applicants also had to present certified evidence of at least five years as a first assistant to a qualified surgeon with no fewer than five hundred major cases, and they had to have performed no fewer than three hundred major surgical cases on their own. In 1929, the category of "fellow" was created to acknowledge doctors with exceptional skill as surgeons and as educators.[6]

In 1939, the ACOS gave its approval to the formation of the American Osteopathic Board of Surgery (AOBS). This board was formed to administer the credentialing and testing of various specialties under the ACOS, including general surgeons, urology, orthopedics, anesthesia, and radiology. The American Osteopathic Academy and the American Osteopathic College of Radiology were both founded in 1941. Today, the AOBS is the certifying board for the following surgical specialties: urology, thoracic-cardiovascular, general vascular, general surgery, neurosurgery, and plastic and reconstructive surgery. All of these surgical disciplines are represented on the certifying board, which remains a committee of the AOA. Certification is recommended by the AOBS, and final approval is decided by the AOA Board of Trustees.[7]

The organization that can claim to be the first osteopathic specialization board was the Eye, Ear, Nose and Throat (EENT) Section of the AOA. Formed in 1908 by a group of EENT doctors practicing at American College of Osteopathic Medicine in Kirksville, Missouri, this organization has evolved over the years to keep abreast of the advances being made in those fields. In 1995, it was renamed American Osteopathic Colleges of Ophthalmology and Otolaryngology–Head and Neck Surgery, and it is comprised of the officers of the individual osteopathic medical colleges. Although the ophthalmologists and the ENT specialists have long since gone their separate ways, the EENT branch of the AOA is still the official organization of these specialists.

In 1927, another group of osteopathic physicians formed their own specialty group, the American College of Osteopathic Internal Medicine. Internists of the time were expected to be up-to-date on cardiology, gastroenterology, oncology, infectious disease, neurology, general medicine, and diagnosis. This was a vast scope of responsibility that required knowledge and expertise in many areas of medicine.

In the office setting, internists' practice was limited to patients referred to them by DO GPs. They offered consultative expertise on the diagnosis and treatment of more complicated medical cases. In the hospital setting, internists served in many capacities: consulting on difficult and challenging cases being managed by the GPs, offering second opinions, co-managing complex post-operative cases, reading and interpreting EKGs, and so on. They were also responsible for training students, interns, and residents in internal medicine. In smaller hospitals, it was not unusual to have one internist on staff with all of these responsibilities while also serving in one capacity or another on the hospital board or as chief of medicine. Today, general internists still play important roles in smaller hospitals and as "hospitalists," managing cases referred to them by GPs and family practice physicians. In larger hospitals, the specialists have taken over and the general internists have been relegated to lesser roles.

In 1934, a group of practicing osteopathic obstetricians met in Wichita, Kansas, and formed the American Association of Osteopathic Obstetrics and Gynecology. At the time and until 1949, their practice was limited to the diseases of females and obstetrics. In 1959, over the objections of the general surgeons, they were finally trained and certified in gynecological surgery. That same year, the American College of Osteopathic Obstetrics and Gynecology was recognized as a separate college by the AOA.[8]

Another key group that has been an essential part of any hospital has been the radiologists. One of earliest X-ray machines in the western United States was at the American School of Osteopathy in Kirksville. The DOs trained in using these devices were early experts in the field. The American College of Osteopathic Radiologists (AOCR) was formed in 1941 and was also under the auspices of the AOA.

By 1945, the AOA had recognized eleven specialty boards.

To meet the demand for ever more medical education and expertise, medical schools and osteopathic medical schools have begun to offer residency programs in family medicine. After an initial rotating internship, family medicine residents continue their studies for an additional two years before certification. The curriculum includes more intensive training in internal medicine, surgery, and obstetrics. At the end of the residency, students are eligible to take an examination to obtain certification in family medicine through the American College of Family Medicine in Family Practice. Some of the MD programs are now proposing a four-year curriculum prior to certification, but so far the osteopathic profession has resisted this trend. Graduates of these programs are very well prepared to practice in today's complex environment; in fact, they are so well trained that they often take positions as hospitalists or emergency room physicians. In Oregon, the residency in family medicine was based at Eastmoreland Hospital in Portland until its closure in 2004.

Osteopathic Specialists in Oregon

From 1917 to 1940, the climate in Oregon for osteopathic specialists was much less welcoming than elsewhere in the country. There were no hospitals available in Oregon for these highly trained osteopathic specialists. Although the laws written in 1917 were finally repealed in 1926, the public perception of DOs' limited scope of practice lingered: no surgery and no prescription of medications. This forbidding climate discouraged DOs from setting up practice in the state. The only osteopathic "specialists" in the state were those "hospital-trained" DO GPs who were trained in some surgery and prescription of medication. In 1930, there were four such hospital-trained DOs in Oregon: Claude Pengra in Portland, Fred Richards in Forest Grove, Manch Gadwa in Salem, and R. R. Sherwood in Medford. In 1930, Pengra was joined by Ira Neher, DO (College of Osteopathic Physicians and Surgeons in Los Angeles 1928).[9]

Neher described his first years in Portland as very difficult. Pharmacists were constantly challenging his prescriptions while the Board of Medical Examiners was trying to prove that he was practicing medicine without a license. Drug company sales representatives (detail men) were not permitted to call on osteopathic physicians. Yet Neher and other DOs persisted, performing surgeries in less-than-optimal hospitals. One such proprietary hospital, City of Roses Hospital owned by Dr. Nicholson, MD, pumped up hospital admissions by allowing Neher to perform surgeries and deliver babies at the hospital, but he would not allow Neher to sign birth certificates or hospital charts. School nurses would not acknowledge his signature on school physicals. With the advent of

WWII, the economy improved and Nicholson began to make it more difficult for Neher and other DOs to admit patients to that hospital.

By 1943, there were enough hospital-trained DOs in the area that serious consideration could be given to forming a separate osteopathic hospital in Portland. With the able assistance of J. C. Long, an insurance executive, three of these DOs came together to form Portland Osteopathic Hospital. Neher, Leonard Purkey, DO, and William Hinds, DO, invested their money to buy an old former hospital/nursing home located at 616 NW 18th Street. Family, friends, patients, and others all pitched in to remodel and otherwise equip this old structure to become a hospital. The hospital opened its doors in May 1944. For the first time, there was an actual osteopathic hospital in Oregon. DO specialists who had long contemplated locating to Oregon now had a place where they could practice their skills.

General surgery, radiology, obstetrics and gynecology, internal medicine, urology, anesthesiology, EENT, and orthopedic surgery all had representation at the facility. DO GPs formed the core of the hospital and provided the preponderance of care, but for the first time they could call on the expertise of DO specialists instead of MDs. With specialists present, the AOA recognized the hospital and approved it for a rotating internship program. The first graduates of the program were Doctors Barr and Wessen (1945–46).

In a short period of time, the hospital was overcrowded. With an active staff of thirty DOs, many coming from outside of Portland, it was time to expand. In 1959, a new thirty-bed hospital opened its doors as Eastmoreland General Hospital. A later addition brought the capacity of the hospital to one hundred beds. In 1973, still another addition was built, which included a fully equipped emergency room, new surgery suites, a modernized lab, and new X-ray facilities.

With these expanded facilities, new, more highly trained DO specialists joined the existing staff, including Charles Woods, pathology; Anthony Cortese, obstetrics and gynecology; Burnham Brooks and Robert Butler, anesthesiology; Philip Cash and Jerry Lancaster, radiology; Richard Turner, internal medicine; and Robert Conley, internal medicine and pulmonology. Edward Heusch, DO, arrived later to provide expertise in hip replacement surgery. Neurology was ably represented by Jon Nelson, and later by A. Paul Aversano.

Most of these specialists relied upon the referrals of DO GPs. During the time these GPs were barred from local MD hospitals, there was plenty of work for all of the specialists. When the MD-dominated hospitals began to woo these DO GPs and their patients, referrals to the osteopathic hospitals and the DO specialists began to wane. New DO specialists found that the welcome at Eastmoreland Hospital was not as cordial, because the referrals that the specialists depended upon came almost exclusively from DO GPs, and there weren't enough referrals to go around.

When MD hospitals began to accept DO specialists onto their staffs, it was possible for DO specialists and sub-specialists to earn a living outside of Eastmoreland Hospital. Rolland O'Dell, DO, was one of the first DO sub-specialists to be accepted at an MD hospital. O'Dell, a highly trained board certified cardiologist, returned to his hometown in Portland intending to practice at Eastmoreland Hospital. Sadly, there was no cardiac catheterization lab or any of the other tools required by a cardiology sub-specialist at Eastmoreland Hospital, so he had to seek privileges at Emanuel Hospital, a local MD hospital. There he was able to team with a cardiac surgeon who was searching for a cardiologist to evaluate his patients prior to open-heart surgery. At first, O'Dell was under intense supervision and scrutiny by the hospital credentials committee, but he quickly established himself as a competent specialist. Later, he was joined by Robert Olson, DO. Together they formed a team that provided excellent care to the cardiology patients admitted to Eastmoreland Hospital while continuing their practice at Emanuel. Later, O'Dell was named Educator of the Year by the students at Emanuel.[10]

As the patient census at Eastmoreland Hospital declined, it became ever more important that DO specialists and sub-specialists reach out to the community and accept referrals from local MDs and other sources, such as local emergency rooms. DOs James Cook, dermatology; Herbert Tirjer, urology; Goeffrey Baum, orthopedics; Charles Kaluza, ENT; Joan Takacs, physiatry; and others all continued to support Eastmoreland Hospital, but were part of the general medical community as well. One of the few DO specialists who derived almost his entire practice from DO referrals was Arthur Rott, board certified in internal medicine, oncology, and hematology. Rott was a much loved and respected educator at Eastmoreland Hospital and many of the DOs he trained remained in the greater Portland area and supported him with referrals.

From its inception, Portland Osteopathic Hospital (later Eastmoreland Hospital) provided an excellent rotating internship program. A loyal and dedicated cadre of specialists and primary care doctors at the hospital provided the education of these interns and, later, the residents in family medicine. Year in and year out, these doctors gave of their time and energy to train these young doctors both in the hospital setting and in their offices.

In 1984, the education committee of the hospital sought and obtained AOA approval to start a family practice residency program. Initially, graduating interns who wished to enter the program were given an additional year of training, following which they were qualified to take the certification exam to became board certified by the American Osteopathic Board of Family Practice. Later, the residency was extended to a three-year program.

By Oregon law, the one-year rotating internship is considered sufficient to allow a graduate to go directly into practice. Initially, most of the graduates of the rotating internship did go directly into practice, but some opted to continue their education by entering a residency in a specialty area. Later, a residency certification became mandatory for any physician to be accepted on the staff of most hospitals. Most insurance companies and their provider panels also required board certification. While the graduates of the rotating internship are licensed by the State of Oregon to practice, the majority of internship graduates enter residencies in other DO or MD specialty programs.

For many years, graduates from the mandatory internship program went directly into practice with another established DO in the area or set up practices on their own. Despite limited resources, Eastmoreland Hospital was instrumental in assisting these new doctors to establish their practices. To assure the success of the freshly minted DOs, the hospital offered assistance with finances, publicity, and patient referrals from the emergency room.

When Eastmoreland Hospital was abruptly closed in 2004 with no advance notice, the residents in training at the time suddenly had no home base. Thanks to the efforts of Residency Director Paula Crone, DO, and the assistance of educators from the College of Osteopathic Medicine in Pomona, California, these trainees were able to complete their training in other parts of the country.

Today, osteopathic primary care physicians and specialists can be found on the medical staffs of nearly every hospital and provider panel in Oregon.

Endnotes

1. Norman Gevitz, *The DOs,* 70
2. Ibid.
3. See biographies of Trostel (page 174), Wood (page 185), and Thiringer (page 172)
4. Ellis Siefer, *A Proud History,* 1
5. Ibid., 4
6. Ibid., 4–10
7. Ibid., 14–17
8. Ibid., 26
9. See Neher biography (page 151)
10. See O'Dell biography (page 154)

CHAPTER 7

Fight for Equality

The privileges now enjoyed by osteopathic physicians are the culmination of a long, uphill battle with the medical establishment. Each step of the way—from the restrictions present in 1907 to the current status of full acceptance—represents a hard-fought battle.

Both nationally and in Oregon, the profession faced powerful opposition by the AMA, OMA, American Hospital Association, the National Pharmacy Association, the insurance industry, and just about every other special interest group that had a stake in maintaining the status quo. In the Oregon state legislature, epic battles were played out in which professional lobbyists employed by the OMA jousted with representative of the OOA. Often, DOs and their patients were instrumental in heading off the attacks of the OMA. Equal practice rights did not come easily.

After numerous battles on the national and state levels, by the 1960s DOs practicing in Oregon had practice privileges very similar to MDs. Most had busy general practices, and if a specialist was required or if the patient needed hospitalization, the patients could be referred to a local osteopathic specialist or hospital. The services of MD specialists were rarely required, but if MD services were required for consultation, the MD would travel to the osteopathic hospital. A large percentage of the DOs practiced in rural areas where they were well received, and because they were located in areas of real need, they were supported legislatively as well.

By the 1960s, the nature of osteopathic medicine practiced by most osteopathic physicians was far different than that practiced in the 1900s. For the most part, they practiced mainstream medicine with osteopathic manipulation relegated to the status of a useful tool. To be sure, there were still DOs who continued to follow the traditional methods. Despite financial success, the struggle to gain acceptance by the medical establishment and the community at large continued. Access to large MD institutions was still barred, the profession was still regarded by the AMA and OMA as a cult, and professional association between MDs and DOs was considered unethical.

The Merger Approach

The fight for full acceptance began in California, where there were nearly 2,000 osteopathic physicians, and disgruntlement with the status of the osteopathic profession was widespread. Many DOs chafed at having to endlessly explain to patients and others: What is an osteopath? Insurance companies provided poor reimbursements, based on the claims that DOs were not as well trained as MDs and therefore deserving of lower reimbursements. In addition, DOs were not able to admit or manage patients in public hospitals and most MD-dominated religious hospitals, and there were limited resources for education at the osteopathic medical schools. Finally, they were tired of being regarded as second-class physicians, both professionally and socially.[1]

For a long time, many DOs and some MDs across the country dreamed of a merger between the medical profession and osteopathy. Yet every time the matter was brought up at AOA meetings, it was soundly defeated. In fact, the California Osteopathic Medical Association was warned that if they persisted in pursuing this path, they risked expulsion from the AOA, but DOs in California continued to pursue this goal despite the warning. Members of the California Medical Association and officers of the California Osteopathic Association created a formal merger proposal in 1961. A survey of the California DOs at the time revealed that six out of seven DOs were in favor of the merger; shortly thereafter, the proposal was approved by the respective associations and then by the general public through a ballot measure.[2]

The merger required several drastic changes in the rules governing DOs. Every DO who wished to obtain an MD license had to pass a simple test, and would then receive an MD diploma. DOs who obtained an MD diploma would no longer be permitted to display their previous DO diplomas. The California College of Osteopathic Medicine would be taken over by an MD school and would no longer issue DO diplomas. (The University of California at Irvine is the result.) All osteopathic training programs throughout the state would be closed, and no new DOs were to be licensed in the state. When the number of DOs who kept their DO diplomas and belonged to the California Osteopathic Association fell below one hundred, the association would be disbanded.[3]

Although the general practitioners were generally happy with their newfound status, the repercussions from the merger were felt locally and nationally. The AOA lost nearly 2,000 members, the number of osteopathic medical schools dropped to five, and the availability of osteopathic rotating internships and training programs was severely diminished. Long-term repercussions were also felt as admissions to small DO hospitals dropped to a point where many had to close their doors. Osteopathic specialists found that their referral base was far smaller than in pre-merger days. Contrary to promises made prior to the merger, DO specialists were learning that it was nearly impossible to gain privileges at many MD hospitals. Medical societies in California continued to bar these "little MDs" from membership.[4]

Merger was considered by at least twelve other state osteopathic associations. In Washington State, a "paper college" was formed and issued a few MD diplomas, but this "college" was soon put out of business by the Washington State Supreme Court. In Oregon, a few DOs traveled to California, and, after taking a simple test, were issued MD diplomas. At the urging of the OMA, the Oregon State Legislature passed legislation forbidding the recognition of the California MD degrees in Oregon. DOs from other states who traveled to California to receive their MD diplomas met the same fate at the hands of their state legislatures.[5]

From the very start of the merger process, a group of loyal DOs in California refused to accept the MD degree. They started a long and uphill battle through the courts to regain status for osteopathic physicians in California. As described earlier, two of the requirements of the merger were that, first, no new DOs would be permitted to practice in the state and, second, when the number of DO members in the California Osteopathic Association fell below one hundred, that organization would be disbanded. To prevent this, many DOs who were of retirement age continued to renew their DO licensure. After a protracted and costly legal struggle, the case was finally settled in 1974 by the California Supreme Court. The court ruled that the merger act unlawfully prohibited new DOs from obtaining licensure as DOs in California.[6]

Over the years, the California example has been used as a cautionary tale whenever the subject of merger is brought up. The concept of two separate but equal professions gained widespread support and is the official policy of the AOA.

Osteopathy and the Military

Another frustrating and humiliating challenge faced by the osteopathic profession was the barring of DOs from serving as military physicians. At the start of WWII, DOs across the country volunteered to serve their country as physicians, but, as in WWI, they were rejected by all the branches of the military. Some volunteered anyway and served their country in other ways. Dr. Charles Carlstrom, for example, served as a major in the quartermaster corps, but as soon as it became known that he was a doctor, he attended servicemen and their families. President Franklin Roosevelt, who had a DO as one of his personal physicians, intervened and made sure that DOs were not drafted into the military. Instead, he advocated for DOs filling the gap left by MDs who had been called up to serve.[7] As a result, DOs across the country established new practices, especially in small towns where they often served as the only doctor in the area. By the end of the war, these doctors had established a cadre of loyal patients who stayed with them even after the MDs returned. George Larson II in Brownsville, A. D. Howells in Albany, David Reid in Lebanon, Larry Jones in Ontario, Bertha Sawyer in Ashland, and many others served their communities with distinction during those years.[8]

During both world wars and the Korean conflict, the ostensible reasoning for barring DOs was that they had insufficient training. In 1963, the U.S. Public Health Service announced that for its purposes, DO and MD degrees would be considered equal. In 1966, it became apparent to Secretary of Defense Robert McNamara that DOs were an important and previously untapped source of primary care physicians. Accordingly, he ordered all branches of the armed forces to accept qualified DOs as physicians and surgeons.[9]

Since that time, DOs have served with distinction in every conflict in which the United States has been involved. Many have risen to high rank, including generals and admirals. At first DOs were used only as primary care physicians, but later, DO specialists were also recruited. Today the United States military has scholarship programs that will pay a substantial portion of the expenses of osteopathic education in exchange for military service after graduation. Since their training emphasizes primary care, DO graduates are considered very desirable by military recruiters.[10]

Endnotes

1. Michael Seffinger, *Resurgence,* 19
2. Norman Gevitz, *The DOs,* 128–132
3. Ibid., 133
4. Michael Seffinger, *Resurgence,* 20
5. Norman Gevitz, *The DOs,* 138
6. Michael Seffinger, *Resurgence,* 24
7. Norman Gevitz, *The DOs,* 113
8. See biographies of Larson (page 141), Howells (page 132), Reid (page 159), and Sawyer (page 166)
9. Norman Gevitz, *The DOs,* 143
10. Michael Seffinger, *Resurgence,* 22

Section Four

Continuing Challenges

CHAPTER 8

The Cost of Health Care

With parity and increased access to hospitals, DOs began to experience the same challenges as MDs. One of the most important was the steadily increasing cost of providing quality health care. There was increasing awareness by the public and their representatives in Congress that the costs for medical care were skyrocketing. New high-tech treatments and diagnostic testing were revolutionizing medical care but the costs were staggering. This led to several efforts to control costs through government intervention and through new models for delivering health care. In addition, the malpractice industry had become far more sophisticated; frequent lawsuits—warranted or not—and huge settlements were driving up the cost of malpractice insurance. These trends have had a profound effect on osteopathic medicine.

Medicare

In 1965, the plight of senior citizens seeking medical care became an important political issue. Legislation creating Medicare and Medicaid as Title XVIII and Title XIX of the Social Security Act was passed by Congress and signed by President Lyndon Johnson, despite strong opposition by the AMA and their state affiliates, the

American Hospital Association, large insurance companies, and other special interest groups on the grounds these programs were "socialized medicine." On the other hand, the AOA supported the concept, but argued that benefits needed to be carefully calibrated to prevent a catastrophic increase in taxation and spending to cover the costs of these programs. Time would prove the AOA position to be correct.[1]

Part A of the new Medicare program provided for the hospital care of millions of Americans over the age of sixty-five. Part B, the voluntary portion of Medicare, would provide medical care for the poor over the age of sixty-five, and for those who desired the coverage and could afford the modest premiums. Medicaid provided care services to low-income children deprived of parental support, their caretaker relatives, the blind, and individuals with disabilities.[2]

Administration of Medicare benefits was the direct responsibility of the federal government, which in turn contracted administration to the large insurance carriers who bid for the business. In the Portland region, Aetna Insurance was the Medicare claims processor. In contrast, Medicaid was administered by the individual states, and the states shared in the overall expense. Eligibility for Medicaid was means-tested, and as a result, there were large disparities in benefits from state to state.

The most immediate effect of Medicare was a dramatic increase in the use of medical services by the covered population. Doctors and hospitals were reimbursed according to the amount billed. Expenses for capital improvements and new facility construction were allowed to be incorporated into the bills submitted by hospitals for patient care. The expenses hospitals incurred as part of their intern and resident training programs were factored in as well. In parts of the country where there were large concentrations of DOs, new hospitals sprang up, and new osteopathic training programs came into existence. While no new osteopathic hospitals were constructed in Oregon, many of the existing hospitals used the Medicare monies to modernize existing facilities and to purchase new and more sophisticated equipment. In Portland, Eastmoreland

Hospital used the money to add a large new addition. For Oregon DOs, an important benefit of Medicare was that there was parity in reimbursements; for the first time, osteopathic physicians did not have to battle to receive equal pay for equal work.[3]

It soon became evident to Medicare administrators and to Congress that Medicare and Medicaid were, financially, a bottomless pit. The monies, which flowed into hospitals, research facilities, and medical education, caused an explosive growth in medical discoveries, technologies, and the specialists ready to use these new discoveries. There was an insatiable demand by the public for the most modern, cutting-edge methods to treat disease. The upside was a dramatic increase in life expectancy from fifty years in 1900 to nearly eighty years today.[4] The downside has been the expenditures required to accomplish this improvement. Clearly something had to be done to control these escalating costs.

Over the years, Congress has passed a series of laws designed to control the costs of medical care for Medicare recipients. Physician standard review organizations (PSROs), physician review organization (PROs), and diagnosis related groups (DRGs) were introduced with the hope that physician review for medical necessity would eliminate the use of tests or surgeries that were of questionable value. The Healthcare Financial Administration (HCFA) and other organizations appeared on the reimbursement scene. These regulators of medicine created whole new bureaucracies that only added more paperwork to the already overburdened physicians and increased the costs of providing care.

Managed Health Care

In 1973, Congress passed The Health Maintenance Organization (HMO) Act. Based on the model of Kaiser and other medical groups, the concept was to deliver health care to HMO members with a prepaid premium designed to cover all of the medical services delivered by the provider members of the plan. Financial risk would be borne by the HMOs, so careful review and approval of all services were required prior to the actual delivery of the service. The HMO provider was expected to emphasize preventive care in the hope of reducing costly medical care. Individual providers were expected to limit expenditures for services because their reimbursements were derived from monies saved when the provider did not order costly tests or procedures. This concept was unpopular with patients and their physicians. Patients often demanded and expected more services than their primary care physician thought necessary, placing doctors in the difficult position of saying "no" to patients who were accustomed to getting what they wanted when they wanted it.[5]

Despite the objections of the medical providers, the HMO concept was popular with employers who wished to provide their employees with health insurance at a reasonable and predictable cost. HMOs seemed to provide a means of controlling the steadily escalating costs of insurance premiums. In Oregon, it was not uncommon for osteopathic physicians to belong to several HMO panels.

The challenge was, and continues to be, the complexity and lack of uniformity of the rules governing HMOs. Some HMOs were quite permissive, while others were very rigid and even arbitrary in their rule enforcement. Individual physicians often joined together in group practices to control the use of surgical procedures, tests, and costly prescriptions, as well as *production* (the number of patients seen per day and the number of charges generated). Local hospitals, desiring a more predictable referral stream, resorted to buying individual practices or small group practices. The formation of an HMO consisting of osteopathic physicians primarily based at Eastmoreland Hospital was contemplated at one point, but had to be rejected because the expense to create such an entity would have been prohibitive and the provider panel would have been too small to be a viable business model.

In 1984, two osteopathic physicians and the current OPSO executive secretary, Jeff Heatherington, created an HMO called FamilyCare Inc. Their goal was to create a managed care organization that provided a comprehensive approach to caring for the underserved

Oregonians on Medicaid. Because of the patient population served and the low reimbursements offered, many Oregon DOs decided not to participate in FamilyCare. Despite the reluctance of many of the primary care DOs, most of the DO specialists supported the program. Thanks to Heatherington's management skills, the Board of Directors, and the loyal support of the doctors who did participate, the HMO has survived and now serves over 50,000 enrollees. To date, it is the only osteopathic HMO in the entire country and the second oldest such organization in Oregon. Excellent management and its nonprofit status have made FamilyCare a successful program financially as well. One of the keys to this HMO's success has been its support of primary care through superior reimbursements and the recognition of the important role of primary care physicians in controlling the overall costs of care.[6]

In 1988, the staff at Eastmoreland Hospital learned that, as of January 1989, Blue Cross/Blue Shield private insurance plans would only deal with HMOs. The Eastmoreland DOs had the choice of joining an HMO that catered to Blue Cross/Blue Shield patients, forming their own HMO, or joining another HMO. Under this threat, the DOs of Eastmoreland Hospital and an MD group from Adventist Hospital joined to form a group called United Healthcare Network (UHN). The principal customer of this HMO was a company called Pacific Care Insurance Company of California. The HMO was contracted to provide medical care and services for Pacific Care's Medicare product Secure Horizons. Using a business model based on the California experience, UHN began to provide medical care for Medicare patients who had purchased this plan. Each provider physician was assigned a panel of patients to manage. Reimbursement was in the form of "capitation" payments which were made to the providers whether the patients were seen or not. Specialty referrals were to be made inside the panel of the specialist providers in UHN. Hospital services were to be provided at Adventist Hospital; Eastmoreland Hospital was not included.

From the very beginning, UHN experienced significant losses. Many of the patients on the plan had serious medical problems that required complex and costly care. Despite the fact that UHN had contracts with other hospitals to provide highly sophisticated services not available at Adventist Hospital, the losses incurred were still enormous. If a patient was referred to an "out of panel" specialist or hospital, the charges were far higher than "in panel." Some of the osteopathic members of the panel had pet specialists to whom they referred, which incurred extra costs to the HMO. Not long after UHN was up and running, Pacific Care launched a recruitment drive in which they offered a "zero premium" feature for their Secure Horizons product. This approach completely defeated the original business model, which was based on a fee of $25 per month to be paid by each patient member.

Despite all of the red ink, UHN continued to operate, hoping the providers would learn to better control costs. Losses were to be borne by both provider groups in the HMO, but during this time, the actual losses were being borne by the Adventist Medical Group of UHN. While the osteopathic providers of the HMO owed similar amounts, they were not being pressured to pay as long as they stayed in UHN. In 2002, UHN was finally dissolved, and the Adventist Group demanded repayment of the debt incurred by the osteopathic members of UHN. It was an enormous sum. After negotiation, each of the DO members was forced to a pay a portion of the debt based on the size of the patient panel he or she managed. In addition, DO providers in this program found that they were sustaining losses caring for these difficult and demanding patients. A loss was incurred each time one of these patients was seen in an individual doctor's office.

Despite all of these cost containment efforts, the cost of medical care in Oregon and across the country has to continue to spiral upwards. Other groups—including Preferred Provider Groups (PPGs), Independent Practice Associations (IPAs), and Physician Hospital Organizations (PHOs)—were introduced, each tasked with saving money. All have failed.

At the present time, the PHO model seems to be dominant.

Hospitals are buying small physician practices and assimilating the doctors into their systems. One of the results of this assimilation has been a decrease in the individual provider's production. Despite this drawback, large physician groups owned and controlled by hospitals are present throughout Oregon.

Another negative effect on production has been the widespread incorporation of Electronic Medical Records (EMR) into medical practice. The positive benefits of EMR are quite profound; however, according to a nationwide survey, the production of individual primary care doctors is reduced by a substantial margin. In addition, patients often complain about the impersonal way physicians interact with them as the physicians enter data into the computer. One solution has been the use of scribes to do the data entry while the physician interacts with the patient. Having to add staff to meet the demands of EMR is another cost multiplier.

Currently, the osteopathic profession is struggling to adjust to the many changes made by the Affordable Care Act on the practice of medicine in general. Another government-induced struggle involves the advent of the medical home model created by Medicare and Medicaid. This model was ostensibly designed to allow patients to access nearly all of their medical needs in one location. The mandated paperwork requirements of this model have forced smaller practices to close and join larger groups. This has been especially burdensome for solo practitioners in small towns.

The Medical Malpractice Crisis

The concept that a learned professional must exercise a reasonable degree of care dates back to the laws of ancient Rome and England, but writings on medical responsibility can be traced back to the Code of Hammurabi of 2030 BC. This code provided that if a doctor treated a patient and that treatment caused the patient to lose an eye or his life, the doctor would have his hands cut off.[7]

Medical malpractice practiced in the United States is derived from English common law and evolved by various rulings in state courts. The legal system is designed to encourage extensive discovery and negotiations between adversarial parties with the goal of resolving the dispute without going to a jury trial.

To claim malpractice, an injured patient must show that the physician acted negligently in rendering care, and that this negligence resulted in injury to the patient. To do so, four legal elements must be proven:

1) a professional duty owed to the patient,
2) a breach of this duty,
3) injury caused to the patient by the breach of duty, and
4) resulting damages incurred by the patient.[8]

Monetary damages, if awarded, typically take into account actual economic loss as well as non-economic loss, such as pain and suffering.

In the United States, medical malpractice suits first appeared in the 1800s; however, legal claims for medical malpractice were rare before the 1960s, and they had little impact on the practice of medicine. Since the 1960s, the frequency of medical malpractice claims has increased. Today, lawsuits filed by aggrieved patients alleging malpractice by physicians or other medical providers and institutions are common. Medical specialists, such as orthopedic surgeons, neurosurgeons, obstetricians, and emergency room physicians, will be sued at least once during their careers.[9] Attorneys specializing in and recruiting aggrieved patients abound. "Expert witnesses" with academic credentials are available, at a price, to testify in nearly every malpractice case, including cases with no merit.

To counter this trend, virtually all physicians began to practice "defensive medicine," where every test and procedure that could be ordered was. The physician's judgment as to whether the test or procedure was actually needed was secondary to the need to practice blameless medicine.

In Oregon, the trend was similar to what was happening around the country. Specialists—who in the course of their specialty are required to perform invasive procedures where the risk of harm is increased—were especially hard hit. Obstetricians and gynecologists, orthopedic surgeons, interventional cardiologists, emergency room physicians, and other specialists found the premiums they were required to pay for malpractice insurance had increased astronomically.

Primary care physicians who cared for low-risk obstetrics patients found their premiums increased, as well as primary care doctors who performed procedures in their offices. In rural areas, pregnant women were forced to travel great distances to find a physician who would care for them.

Most of the osteopathic physicians in Oregon were GPs who provided primary care, and many of these DOs practiced in small towns in rural Oregon where they were the only doctor in town. These doctors were especially hard hit by increases in malpractice insurance premiums. Since they were the only doctors in these small towns, it was important that they continue to provide a full spectrum of care to the people of their communities. It was also critical for these rural doctors to keep their service prices to a minimum because so many of their patients had no insurance and paid cash for medical treatment. Many of these doctors purchased malpractice insurance and "ate" the difference in costs, obviously decreasing their income.

Some physicians—those who were already operating their practices on a thin margin—opted to "go bare." They made it clear to their patients that they had no malpractice coverage, yet the loyal townspeople continue to support them. The strategy of "going bare" was not condoned by hospitals. Most hospitals required documentation that the physicians on staff or applying for staff privileges were covered.

Initially, the minimum required coverage for a GP was $300,000 maximum per event and $600,000 cumulative maximum; as time progressed, these coverage minimums were increased to $1,000,000 and $3,000,000 respectively. For specialists, the required coverage minimum was millions of dollars more, and premiums for certain "high risk" specialties could be in excess of $100,000 per year.[10] With all of the potential for human error that can be found in the operation of a hospital, one can imagine the premiums paid by hospitals. Little wonder that the price for an office visit, a procedure, or a hospital stay has risen so dramatically.

For many years, DOs could purchase their malpractice insurance through an agency in California, Chubb Indemnity Group. The premiums were quite stable for many years, but in the 1970s, the malpractice suit epidemic and some huge awards caused the company to cancel malpractice insurance for every DO in Oregon.

There was a grace period during which DOs could search for other insurance coverage. Professional Mutual Insurance Company, a company based in Kansas City, Missouri, was licensed in Oregon to write malpractice insurance. This company catered to the needs of the osteopathic physicians, but it was unfortunately unable to underwrite the osteopathic specialists in the state. This dilemma hit the specialists practicing at Eastmoreland Hospital especially hard. They were loyal DOs who practiced almost exclusively at Eastmoreland Hospital and primarily consulted and treated patients referred by osteopathic primary care doctors. These DO specialists also played a very important role in the postgraduate training of DO students and interns. With the risk of malpractice suits an everyday concern, none of these specialists were willing to accept the risk of financial ruin by "going bare." In addition, the hospital faced the risk of these specialists moving elsewhere and the resultant rapid financial deterioration that would occur if these specialists were not on the job.

One of the anesthesiologists at the hospital, Robert Butler, DO, took the politically courageous step of approaching the "archenemy"—the Oregon Medical Association. He learned that if the DOs who needed malpractice coverage would join the OMA, they would be eligible to purchase malpractice insurance through CNA Insurance Company. Despite the risk of alienating their DO referral base, these DOs did join the OMA and soon had malpractice coverage.

Backlash from the OOA and AOA came swiftly. The specialists were reprimanded and, to this day, are no longer members of the OOA. However, the local DOs who referred to these specialists supported them totally.

Coverage by Professional Mutual Insurance Company soon became problematic as the company began to experience unsustainable losses. In 1986, the company went into receivership and had to cancel their Oregon policies, and the DOs were again looking for coverage. Happily, a local company, Northwest Physicians Mutual Company, was just forming. They were happy to underwrite the DO GPs in Oregon, and OMA membership was not required. Today the company has combined with another malpractice company in California called The Doctors Company. For now, at least, malpractice coverage for Oregon DOs and DO specialists is assured.

As the costs to the medical system have escalated, numerous attempts have been made to rein in malpractice insurance costs. A host of strategies have been introduced in state legislatures across the country. So far, these attempts to make the system fairer and less costly for physicians and their patients have been successfully opposed by the trial lawyers across the country. Perhaps the advent of the Affordable Care Act will force meaningful reforms.

Endnotes

1. Norman Gevitz, *The DOs,* 155
2. Ibid.
3. Ibid., 157
4. U.S. Census 2010
5. Norman Gevitz, *The DOs,* 159
6. See J. Scott Heatherington biography (page 120)

7. B. Sonny Bal, *An Introduction to Medical Malpractice in the United States,* 1
8. Ibid., 6
9. Ibid., 10
10. Professional Mutual Insurance Company, Kansas City, Missouri

CHAPTER 9

Osteopathic Manipulation Therapy

One of the distinguishing practices of osteopathy—and one of its most controversial aspects—is the use of osteopathic manipulation therapy (OMT). The term was coined by A. T. Still.[1] He taught that osteopathic manipulation adjusted the spine in a way that removed obstructions to blood flow, lymphatic flow, and neurological function. Once these obstructions were removed, the body could resume normal functioning. When a manual examination revealed an area of increased temperature, increased moisture, or a subtle yet detectable area of restricted motion, that area would be treated with massage, manipulation, or both.

A method of manipulation called *high velocity, low amplitude* consisted of rapidly increasing the flexion/extension or rotation of the identified spinal area. Usually a popping sound would result, and the patient often experienced sudden relief of the symptoms. Still taught that a large spectrum of diseases could be treated in this manner, including asthma, and it was highly effective in relieving the symptoms of back pain, especially back strains. The high velocity, low amplitude method was also applied to the extremities. In an era when manual labor was the norm, a method that would treat pain and get the worker back on the job was very popular.

Most osteopathic physicians were perfectly happy to incorporate Still's mechanistic explanations on exactly how OMT worked.

The fact that it did work and helped their patients was enough. Louisa Burns, DO, of the Pacific College of Osteopathic Medicine, set about to discover exactly what happens when OMT was used. Her research conducted on animals prior to WWI was thought to demonstrate that there was a correlation between spinal findings and certain diseases in the lab animals.[2]

Her findings were largely discredited, but between 1941 and 1943, J. Stedman Denslow, DO, and Irwin M. Korr, PhD, published research articles demonstrating that conditions in other parts of the body produced reflex spasms in the spinal musculature that were isolated to one or two spinal segments. They further demonstrated that stimulated or spasmodic segments in the spine could produce symptoms in other parts of the body,[3] hence the term *spinal lesion.* Spinal lesions could be detected by palpation and relieved by OMT. Later, the term *somatic dysfunction* was introduced to describe an area that would require treatment.

By its very nature, high velocity OMT is sometimes difficult to administer, and can be painful or alarming to the patient. Very large patients, children, or elderly patients required careful treatment. Despite this, actual injuries to the spine through OMT were exceedingly rare.

In 1939, William Garner Sutherland, DO, wrote and self-published a volume entitled *The Cranial Bowl.* In this work, Sutherland described a rhythm associated with breathing that produces subtle motions of both the cranial bones and the sacrum.[4] By applying gentle pressure to the bones of the skull and to the sacrum, various conditions—including epilepsy, migraine, depression, and the like—could be treated. Viola Freyman, DO, incorporated these methods at her Osteopathic Center for Children and Families in San Diego, successfully treating children with brain damage and severe disabilities.[5]

Other OMT methods followed, including the Myofascial Release Method. Myofascial Release is used to treat somatic dysfunction and the resultant pain and motion restriction. Treatment consists of continual feedback through palpation and gentle application of tractive or rotational forces to restore normal motion and physiologic function.[6]

In 1948, Fred Mitchell, DO, developed a method called the Muscle Energy technique. This technique is a direct and active technique. The operator identifies a *restrictive barrier,* and the patient is asked to exert his muscles in the direction opposite to the barrier. By doing so, the muscles forming the barrier relax. This method has long been popular with DOs, and has also been incorporated by many other practitioners, including physical therapists, rehabilitation therapists, and chiropractors. It is an effective technique that is simple to apply.[7]

In 1955, Lawrence Jones, DO, of Ontario, Oregon, began to publish articles about a method of manipulation he termed *counterstrain.* This treatment method involves identifying a tender point that correlates with the area of motion restriction. Correction occurs by positioning the tender area until the tenderness disappears or lessens and then holding that position for ninety seconds. Today, this method is the primary method taught by many colleges of osteopathic medicine.[8]

In A. T. Still's day, the only OMT method available was the high velocity, low amplitude method. Today, the osteopathic physician can offer the patient a full knowledge of medicine plus the ability to diagnose and treat problems amenable to OMT. They are trained in a variety of OMT methods and can use these methods and others in combinations to suit the gender, size, and age of the patient.

Research into the physiology of OMT has been difficult. Unlike a double-blind study testing the efficacy of a medication, no one has developed a method where the patient, much less the doctor, does not know that a treatment is taking place. Despite these challenges, research continues, and there is a continued search for an explanation of exactly how and why OMT is effective, particularly an explanation that can be categorized as *evidence-based medicine.*

Despite the fact that innumerable patients have been benefited from OMT, it is still not recognized by many insurance companies, and reimbursement for the time and effort required to administer an osteopathic treatment has lagged far behind reimbursement for other procedures. For this reason, busy DOs will often forego the administration of OMT. Despite this limitation, younger DOs searching for an alternative to mainstream medicine have found that it is indeed a highly effective method that patients appreciate.

Endnotes

1. Norman Gevitz, *The DOs,* 21
2. Ibid., 62–63
3. Ibid., 104–106
4. Sutherland Society, "General Information on Cranial Osteopathy"
5. Michael A. Seffinger, *Resurgence,* 111
6. Wikipedia, "Osteopathic manipulative medicine"
7. Wikipedia, "Muscle energy technique"
8. See Jones biography (page 136)

CHAPTER 10

Osteopathic Education in Oregon

For the osteopathic profession to survive and grow, education opportunities, both through osteopathic medical schools and through internship and residency openings, are critical. During the 1970s, the rapid loss of osteopathic hospitals as training sites for future osteopathic specialists and primary care doctors would have seemed to indicate the outlook for the future of the osteopathic profession was bleak indeed. But in reality, the situation was quite the opposite. Osteopathic hospitals taken over by MD-dominated organizations or corporations continued to be staffed by cadres of DOs who carried on their osteopathic training programs. The AOA soon certified these hospitals and expanded opportunities by accepting training programs in other hospitals where the staff was dominated by MDs. As a result, the number of training slots available to osteopathic students was actually increased.[1]

In 1969, the first new osteopathic medical school in fifty years was opened at Michigan State University. This school was partially funded by the State of Michigan and was soon followed in rapid succession by new osteopathic medical schools in Texas (1970), Oklahoma (1974), West Virginia (1974), Ohio (1975), New Jersey and New York (1977), New England (1978), and California (1978). Since these osteopathic schools were founded, many more have been added. Some of these schools received state funding, but most have relied on tuition to fund their programs. As a result, twenty percent of all freshmen who entered any medical school in 2013 were osteopathic medical students.[2]

In 1978, the College of Osteopathic Medicine of the Pacific (COMP) was formed in Pomona, California. Under the able leadership of Philip Pomeranz, PhD, and his board, the school has grown to become Western University of Health Sciences. In addition to the osteopathic medical school, there are eight additional colleges devoted to allied health sciences. The presence of this medical school and its graduates has revitalized the osteopathic medical community in California and in the neighboring states of Oregon and Washington.[3]

While Oregon law regulating the osteopathic profession required that a DO serve a one-year rotating internship, insurance plans and hospitals were beginning to require that all physicians who wished to be on hospital staff or be reimbursed for their services be board certified. In 1984, the education committee of Eastmoreland Hospital, working with the education committee of the AOA, created a family medicine residency based at Eastmoreland Hospital. The program was designed to be a three-year program. The first class had already served a one-year internship, so after another two years of training, the first group of residents graduated in 1986 and were board eligible to take the certification exams for the American College of Family Practice.

Initially, some of the young doctors in training opted to go into practice after serving the one-year rotating internship required by the AOA. At the same time, DO GPs who were already in practice were permitted to take certification examinations and were also certified by the American College of Osteopathic Family Physicians. The MDs were also offering residencies in family practice, and, like the DOs, offered certification to GPs who wished to be board certified by the American Academy of Family Practice. Because of the interest in sub-specialty training programs by young MD graduates, the slots in allopathic family practice residencies had been going unfilled and were made available to DO students.

From its inception, the residency program at Eastmoreland was a source of excellent primary care physicians serving Oregon and the Pacific Northwest. Happily, many have chosen to remain in Oregon, often in the greater Portland area. Thanks to a loyal cadre of specialists and GPs, the residency program was widely recognized for the quality of its medical education. Under the able leadership of several doctors, including Dr. Tony Smith and later Dr. Paula Crone, the residents had outpatient care opportunities at clinics sponsored by FamilyCare Inc. When the patient census at Eastmoreland Hospital decreased, patient experience and clinical training were made available to DO residents at several of the MD-dominated hospitals in the area.

In 1995, the AOA created a consortium called Osteopathic Postdoctoral Training Institutions (OPTI), which attempted to accredit all hospitals offering postgraduate medical training, whether osteopathic or allopathic.

In 2003, with the assistance of the administrative staff of OPSO, Eastmoreland Hospital, and the leadership of Dirk Foley, a new educational program for third- and fourth-year students from the Northwest was created. The program was called the Northwest Track (NWT) and thirty third- and fourth-year students from the Pomona school came to Oregon to serve their clerkship requirements. Several graduates from the NWT and COMP served internships and family practice residencies at Eastmoreland Hospital.[4]

In 2009, Jeff Heatherington, CEO of FamilyCare Inc. and executive secretary of OPSO, met with Larry Mullins, CEO of The Samaritan Hospital Group, a five-hospital group with 250 physician providers headquartered in Lebanon, Oregon. Initially, this was to be a one-hour meeting to discuss possible residency slots for osteopathic postgraduates in the OPTI model. What followed was a conversation that lasted the entire morning. Both the men were inspired by the possibility of constructing an osteopathic medical school in Lebanon. Samaritan had been granted a fifty-acre plot of land directly across the street from the hospital in Lebanon, and Mullins and his board of directors had dreamed of using this land to create a medical complex to serve the people of Lebanon, as well as the entire Northwest. Heatherington put forward the idea that the medical school would be an ideal culmination of that dream. In short order, Heatherington contacted COMP to ask if they would be interested in creating a branch campus in Lebanon, and Mullins took the idea to the board of directors of the Samaritan Hospital Group.

Not long afterward, the board of directors and trustees of COMP met and approved the funding of feasibility studies for the formation of the new school. Dr. Ben Cohen of COMP then contacted Bill Bryan, PhD, a retired educator who had been instrumental in forming three new osteopathic medical schools in various parts of the country. Although Bryan made his headquarters in Florida, he began a series of trips to the Lebanon area and to Portland during which he exhaustively researched the feasibility of an osteopathic medical school in Lebanon. He met with nearly every businessperson in the city and found strong support for the concept of the school. The Mayor, the City Council, the Chamber of Commerce, and others were excited by the idea of a medical school in their city, which had nearly been destroyed in the 1990s by the curtailing of the timber industry to save the spotted owl. Bryan also traveled around Oregon to seek support for the idea, and he found strong support in the osteopathic medical community.

After Bryan's report, COMP, in conjunction with the AOA, put in motion plans to form the new school. While Bryan was building support in the community of Lebanon, Mullins moved ahead with the actual construction process. Plans were drawn up and soon a new building was rising.

The recruitment process for the dean of the new school was already under way during construction. Dr. Paula Crone, a graduate of COMP and the family practice residency program at Eastmoreland Hospital, accepted the challenge as dean of the new school.

Planning for the curriculum, faculty, and staff for the new College of Osteopathic Medicine Northwest (COMP-Northwest) began under the able guidance and advice of Clint Adams, DO (dean of the Pomona school), Bryan, and other leaders. The plan was to follow the curriculum already established at Pomona, but the selection of faculty and staff was Crone's responsibility. Early in the planning and recruiting process, the school was headquartered in the same offices as OPSO in Portland. This served as the hub for the all-important fundraising effort that would help to defray the costs of this undertaking. David Walls and the board of OPSO frequently collaborated with the staff of COMP-Northwest to create a successful osteopathic medical school in Oregon. Later, the temporary headquarters were moved to a hospital-owned clinic building in Lebanon. The goal was to open the school in 2011. Students began to apply and were initially interviewed in rooms at Samaritan Hospital.

The initial "White Coat" ceremony was held on a hot July day in 2011. There were no facilities in Lebanon large enough to accommodate the anticipated crowd, so a huge tent was erected in the parking lot of the new school. Dignitaries from California and the local area attended, along with families and friends of the new medical students. The ceremony was presided over by Deans Crone and Adams. Governor Kitzhaber of Oregon gave a speech about the future of medicine and the role that primary care physicians must play in the future care of the people of Oregon and the United States. Dean Crone challenged the students and professors to make COMP-Northwest the best osteopathic medical school in the country.

Currently, the students of the class of 2015 have embarked on their clinical rotations and have met with an overwhelmingly positive reception by the preceptors that will be training them prior to their graduation as DOs. The future is bright indeed!

Endnotes

1. Norman Gevitz, *The DOs,* 183
2. Dirk Foley, "The Northwest Track Origins," *COMP Northwesterly,* 1
3. Michael A. Seffinger, *Resurgence,* 55
4. Dirk Foley, "The Northwest Track Origins," *COMP Northwesterly,* 2

Section Five

The People

CHAPTER 11

The People

Over the last several years, I have interviewed many retired Oregon osteopathic physicians and lay persons who have supported the profession. The biographies compiled in this section are based on those interviews. These men and women have played an influential part in the osteopathic profession; some have quietly and faithfully served their local communities in both medical and civic capacities, while others have had an influence felt regionally, nationally, and even internationally. Many have already been mentioned in this book; all have been a credit to their profession. Here are their stories.

John Aaronson, DO 1922 – 2014

One of the enjoyable aspects of this history project has been getting acquainted with and listening to the stories of the DOs who practiced outside Portland. I recently interviewed Dr. Aaronson and his wife Carol at their home in Myrtle Creek, Oregon. Aaronson is a lively ninety-year-old, still practicing osteopathic manipulation therapy (OMT) once a week at nearby Canyonville, and every other week in Central Point. This is his story.

Aaronson was born into an osteopathic family in California; his father, a Kirksville graduate, worked until he was eighty-four, then shortly thereafter passed away. Aaronson entered the University of California but "flunked out." Shortly afterward, he was drafted into the U.S. Navy as a corpsman. He was shipped to Hawaii and was scheduled to enter the war at Guam. Because he was quite proficient with paperwork, he instead became a clerk and stayed in Hawaii. The rest of his unit shipped for Guam, where most of the men he trained with lost their lives.

He was then approached and asked if he would like to become a doctor. Aaronson said he spent the night deliberating; in the morning he said "yes." He was then sent to Gonzaga University to complete his premed education. While there, his skill as a trumpeter allowed him to form a band that was so good they had a weekly radio broadcast playing dance music.

After completing his premed classes, he was accepted at the Medical College of Virginia to be trained as an MD. WWII had ended, so he transferred to Kirksville College of Osteopathy as soon as he could, graduating in 1949.

He interned at Burbank Osteopathic Hospital in California and it was here that he began his career as an anesthesiologist. His trainers got him started administering anesthesia, and once he became proficient, the attending doctors would leave the hospital, turning the responsibilities over to Aaronson. He also had all of the usual responsibilities of a DO intern in those days, which was everything or anything that might happen in the hospital while the intern was on duty.

After completing his internship, he decided to locate in Milwaukie, Oregon. He practiced there for a brief time until he injured his back while constructing his own clinic building. He needed surgery, so he returned to Burbank and had the required procedure.

During his recovery, he was contacted by Weldin Falk, DO, who had a practice and hospital in Canyonville, Oregon. When Aaronson arrived in Canyonville, Falk informed him that he would be in charge for the next month. During that month, he delivered babies, set bones, and attended injured loggers. He even had to perform an emergency appendectomy, something he had seen performed but had never done. (One hears the old adage "see one, do one, teach one" mentioned in the process of training young doctors, but until now I always thought it was some kind of legend.) He didn't have an anesthesiologist present, so one of the operating room nurses gave the anesthetic under Aaronson's supervision—the patient lived! As was typical for the times, in addition to his surgical duties, he would see on average sixty patients a day.

He served in Canyonville from 1952 to 1967. In addition to his duties as house anesthesiologist for Falk, he enjoyed obstetrics and delivered an estimated 2,000 babies. Along with his medical duties, he served on the school board, was the team physician for the local high school football team, and was active in the Oregon Osteopathic Association, including a term as president.

Following his work at Canyonville, he and his second wife Carol moved back to Los Angeles, where he practiced anesthesiology almost exclusively. When time permitted, he also continued his work as a GP and continued to play his trumpet.

Not long after their daughter was born, he witnessed an altercation on a Los Angeles freeway which convinced him to leave the area at once. Coincidently, that very night he received a call from Max Flowers, DO, in Central Point, Oregon, asking if he would be interested in a position at Crater General Hospital. It didn't take the family long to move to Central Point, and Aaronson worked as a GP and anesthesiologist the hospital there until 1994.

To enhance his skills he often took courses in various subjects, such as a manipulation course in Arizona, and a cardiology course with emphasis on interpretation of EKGs in Chicago. He also invited prospective medical students to "shadow" him while he saw his patients.

He retired in 1994, and he and his wife built their dream home in the little town of Myrtle Creek. He "unretired" shortly thereafter and practiced with a nurse practitioner, providing OMT skills and GP work. After six years, he slowed down to his present pace.

When asked what was the most rewarding part of his career as an osteopathic physician, he stated that the satisfaction of being able to help nearly all of his patients in one way or another. OMT often provided instant results that were very much appreciated. His biggest disappointment was when he had to stop his general medical practice. If he could he would still be working full time.

His advice to young doctors: "Go for it! Learn OMT well, because it is a very rewarding and unique service you can offer your patients."

Paul Aversano, DO 1947 –

As I have interviewed DOs over the past several years, it is clear that certain individual DOs have made important contributions to the establishment of an osteopathic medical school in Oregon. Some have contributed by earning the trust of their patients, thereby creating positive influences in the political arena. Most have made a difference in the communities they served. Many have served as mentors to students in their medical offices; others as consultants and educators in the hospital setting. Paul Aversano is that rare clinician who has managed to fill all these roles and continues to contribute as an educator at the new osteopathic medical school in Lebanon.

Born in Buffalo, New York, Aversano was raised in a family that placed a high premium on education. His father was a manager/chemist at a local pharmaceutical company, and his mother was a dedicated homemaker who created a home atmosphere that encouraged intellectual pursuits. Both Aversano and his sisters were educated in private schools. In addition to his studies, he excelled in baseball and other sports. At times, Aversano found it difficult to concentrate on his studies and still participate in sports, but his parents made sure that he could do both.

At an early age, Aversano decided he wanted to be a doctor. When he mentioned this to the headmaster of his school, he was advised that he would never make it. After high school, he decided to attend Washington and Jefferson College where he could pursue his interests in baseball and science. His passion was biology.

After graduation, he applied for medical school in the New York area. A fellow student told him about DO schools, so Aversano thought he would apply. One of the requirements for application was a reference from a DO. He had to travel through a snowstorm to Erie, Pennsylvania, to get to the DO he would shadow. The doctor was very gracious and allowed him to see his patients on hospital rounds.

He had his interview at the DO medical school in Des Moines, Iowa. When asked the difference between an allopath and an osteopath, he answered he didn't have a clue. At the end of the interview, a young doctor (the actual dean of the school) at the interview asked him what would make him decide which medical school to attend. Aversano replied, "Whichever one picks me first!" Happily, he opted for an osteopathic education.

He spent the last six months of his training working with John Nelson, DO, a neurologist at Portland Osteopathic Hospital in Oregon. He said he fell in love with Oregon after seeing a TV series featuring the state. He graduated from Des Moines in 1973, and did a rotating internship at Brentwood Hospital in Cleveland, Ohio. He followed this with a residency at the famed Cleveland Clinic, completing his training program in 1977.

There was already a place for him to practice in Portland, so he went to work not long after completing his residency. He soon found himself with a busy practice, consulting, managing hospital patients, and training students and interns. In addition, he took on the responsibilities of Director of Medical Education, Chief of Staff, and participant on other committees.

In 1978, he was recruited by and began to teach neurology at the new College of Osteopathic Medicine (COMP) in Pomona, California. He would fly to Los Angeles, teach for five days in a row, then return to his responsibilities in Portland.

After five years, Nelson left the practice, leaving Aversano with the responsibility of all the neurologic cases at Eastmoreland Hospital. During this time, Aversano also coordinated the placement of students from COMP and other osteopathic medical schools in offices around the Portland area. Despite this frantic schedule, he found the time to pursue golf, and, due to his athletic ability, became a very good golfer.

He was so busy that he ignored his developing cancer symptoms. When he finally sought treatment, he learned that he would have a prolonged recovery and he was forced to retire from his practice. It was during this period that his marriage of seventeen years came to an end. Despite these setbacks, he continued to consult, lecture, and assist in coordinating externships.

In August of 2003, he married Paula Crone, DO, a local family practice doctor that he had helped to train. For a time they continued their separate practices. In addition to her busy family practice, Crone was in charge of the Family Practice Residency program at Eastmoreland Hospital. The success of this program soon attracted attention from around the country. With their combined expertise in medical education, the couple was called upon to help form residency training programs in Corvallis, Oregon.

Shortly thereafter, plans began for the development of an osteopathic medical school in Oregon. After the location was selected, personnel from the Samaritan Hospital Group (headquartered in Lebanon, Oregon) and the Pomona school combined their expertise and the ball was rolling. They interviewed a few candidates for the dean's position, but the interviewing committee unanimously agreed that Crone was the right person. It quickly became apparent that they had hired a Dean Team.

Today, in addition to teaching neurology, Aversano fills many roles as backup for Dean Crone. Aversano wholeheartedly supports

Crone's goal for the school—preparing young people to become the best osteopathic family physicians in the world.

Aversano says his greatest satisfaction has been the privilege of caring for his patients, to be involved in their lives and make a difference. His greatest disappointment was the loss of Eastmoreland Hospital and the wonderful atmosphere it embodied.

He is very optimistic about the future of the osteopathic profession. His advice to young people considering entering the profession: Enter with your eyes open. It is not an easy road; it will require a minimum of seven years of hard work to attain the goal, but in the end, it is well worth it.

John Bauers, DO 1925 – 1998

After WWII, a large number of refugees/displaced persons (DPs) from Europe who had to leave their homes came to the United States to seek employment and a new life. Many of these people were highly educated and skilled in specialties that were in short supply in the United States. Some became osteopathic physicians and the profession benefited greatly from their presence. One such immigrant was Dr. John Bauers, who was my medical partner for many years. This is his story as related by his daughters Dana and Liz, son John, family friend Lynn, nephew Ivars, and through audio recordings of his mother Elizabeth, sister Liga, and Aunt Erna.

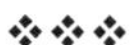

John Bauers, whose birthname was Janis (pronounced "Ya-niss"), was born in Ranka, Latvia, in 1925 to Ernest Bauers, minister of agriculture for Latvia (1923 through 1924), and his mother Elizabete Brants Bauers, a schoolteacher and homemaker. On November 18, 1918, Ernest Bauers was a member of the Latvian Parliament, which proclaimed Latvia's independence on that day. Janis' father passed away at the age of forty-four from endocarditis when Janis was only a year old.

Janis and his older sister Liga were raised by their mother on an 87-acre farm, devoted to raising fruits, vegetables, and a few farm animals for their personal consumption. Much of the farm was rented to others who raised wheat and rye. The family homestead was named *Kalnietis*, which means "people who live on the mountain." The Kalnietis property included some forestland where Janis, his sister, and his mother picked mushrooms and berries, and the Gauja River where Janis swam and fished as a boy.

Janis' paternal grandfather, Pavels Bauers, had purchased this land from German barons in 1872, making periodic payments in gold Russian rubles, the preferred currency in that era. Pavels Bauers raised flax, rye, and wheat, which he sold to make payments on his 250-acre farm, which also included the Kalnietis farm where Janis grew up.

Janis' maternal grandfather, Georgs Brants, owned a farm and winery about forty miles to the north, and was known to make and sell excellent wine made from fruit and berries, something that would interest Janis later in life.

Janis' early education was in the public school system at the elementary school in Reveli (near Ranka), walking distance from home, and continued even during the years of WWII. When Latvia was occupied by the Soviet Union in June 1940, they came into Janis' high school in Cesis, Latvia, and arrested a classmate who had apparently spoken out against the Russians. He was never seen again.

A year later, on June 14, 1941, Soviet soldiers rounded up 40,000 Latvians who were on a blacklist and sent them to Siberia by rail in cattle cars. Janis' mother learned that they, along with other family members, were on a second blacklist for deportation to Siberia, probably because her husband had been a government official. The second deportation to Siberia never occurred. Nazi Germany attacked the Soviet Union, and the German army occupied Latvia on July 1, 1941, driving out the Soviet army. During the years of German occupation, Janis and his family continued to live on their farm. His mother recalled she had to hide their food in their forest when German soldiers came looking for food supplies for their army.

The Soviet army re-entered Latvia in July 1944 and began to drive out the German army. In September of that year, the German army strongly recommended everyone leave their homes in the area where nineteen-year-old Janis lived with his family. The only option to leaving was hiding somewhere until the German army left. Mother Bauers decided that the family and their housekeeper, Ieva, should leave for their own safety, so they packed their horse-drawn wagon with sacks of flour, food, clothing, and other supplies, and began the 200-mile journey to the port of Liepaja in southern Latvia. Not wanting to leave the few cows and sheep behind, they took them along.

They buried some of their more valuable belongings, thinking they would surely be returning home in a few weeks. On their way they stopped in Riga, where Elizabeth's 74-year-old mother, her three sisters, her sister Erna's small children (four and two years old), and Erna's husband joined them. Elizabeth's brother Juris, who was a manager at in the Latvian State Alcohol Factory, gave her a number of bottles of alcohol similar to Everclear for the journey. Elizabeth said these bottles of alcohol would prove to be very valuable during their journey because they could use them like money.

According to Elizabeth, the roads were full of people evacuating the country along with the German army. Since most German young men were in the army, Germany needed farm workers and other laborers, and they hoped the people evacuating Latvia and the other Baltic States would help fill this need. About 150,000 Latvians were evacuated to Germany in this way.

Janis' mother recalls that they walked during the day and rested through the night to stay ahead of the Soviet army. They slept under the stars and in abandoned homes, and when they had a chance, baked bread along the way. Sometimes they were turned away by farmers who wouldn't let them sleep in their barn. When they woke up in the morning, they could often hear the sound of battle, often in the direction they had to travel. At one point, the German army transported them for a few miles in exchange for some bottles of the alcohol Elizabeth's brother had given to her.

They were able to reach the Latvian seaport city of Liepaja after about a month on the road. They spent about three days in Liepaja before boarding a ship that would take them to the port of Danzig (now Gdansk), Poland. The Soviet Air Force often dropped bombs in an attempt to stop these ships full of refugees. When they reached Danzig, they boarded a train for the 380-mile journey to the city of Gorlitz, just a few miles inside Germany. These trains were in the crosshairs of the Soviet Air Force, but fortunately their train wasn't bombed.

In an area known as Niederschlesien, in the vicinity of Gorlitz, they found jobs on a dairy farm with the help of the local burgermeister (mayor). The women helped make butter, cream, and cheese. Elizabeth recalled that Janis, at the time in poor health with tuberculosis contracted from an uncle, was required to work very hard, digging a well when it was very cold and carrying containers of coal for heating the dairy up a steep ladder.

It wasn't long before the Soviet army was about to enter Germany. With the army rapidly approaching, the Bauers' family was once again given warning by German government officials to flee for their safety. Not knowing what to do, they turned to the local burgermeister, who found a farmer to take them to the train station in Gorlitz. They found a supervisor at the train station who was willing to let them stay at his place until there was a train available bound for Bavaria in southern Germany. They were awakened during the night two days later, and told they could board a train first thing in the morning for Bavaria.

In Bavaria, a local farmer gave them refuge and they worked there until the American army entered at the end of the war in May 1945. An American tank with a few soldiers rolled onto the farm and a couple of warning shots were fired into the air. The farmer's wife had hung white bed sheets out the windows prior to the Army's arrival to indicate they were not a threat. When the American soldiers spotted Janis, they immediately thought he was a German soldier because of his age. They took him into temporary custody and put him on their tank, but the family succeeded in convincing the soldiers Janis was a Latvian displaced person, not a German soldier.

The American army set up various displaced person (DP) camps in Bavaria, and the first DP camp where the family stayed was in former German army housing somewhere not far from the farm where they had been working. From there they and other DPs were fortunate enough to stay in a resort located in Streitberg for several months. Eventually they ended up in a DP camp in the city of Erlangen, which was located north of Nuremberg in the American Zone in Germany. While residing in the camp, Janis was able to enroll in university and embarked on science studies.

Janis had been living with tuberculosis for some time, and he needed treatment in a hospital. He eventually had to have a portion of his lung removed before he was pronounced fit to emigrate. In preparation for Janis' surgery, his mother had obtained a small supply of penicillin from relatives in Sweden, but this wasn't enough to treat him after surgery. His mother then sought help from the American army, and she obtained additional penicillin for Janis to avoid infection and survive the surgery. It was during his stay in the hospital he decided he wanted to be a doctor.

The American officials asked the family and other Latvian DPs if they wanted to return to Latvia, not knowing the danger and risk of deportation to Siberia that awaited anyone who returned to the Soviet-occupied country. Latvian DPs eventually ended up in various parts of the world, but the Bauers knew they wanted to live in America. Family members and other emigrants found American sponsors and left the camp for the New World. The Bauers had to delay their departure to allow treatment of Janis' tuberculosis so he could receive the clean bill of health he needed to enable him to enter America.

Finally, in June 1950, Janis and his mother were able to come to America and it was then that Janis Bauers officially became John Bauers. They entered the country in New Orleans, and with the sponsorship of both a local family and the First English Lutheran Church in St. Joseph, Missouri, they settled there. Elizabeth immediately began working as a housekeeper and cook for the family that sponsored them at a starting salary of $15 per week.

John lived for a while on a farm not far from St. Joseph where his sister Liga and brother-in-law were working. The farm was owned by the family that employed his mother. The small farmhouse where the Bauers family lived had no electricity or running water, and was heated with a wood stove. His first job was cooking hamburgers in a small diner. Later he worked as a radiology technician at the hospital in St. Joseph.

From the outset, it must have been evident that this very bright young man was capable of far more than a career as an X-ray tech, and he was urged by the chief of radiology to go into medicine. He applied for medical school, and was accepted in 1954 into the Kansas City College of Osteopathic Medicine in Missouri.

John arrived in the United States fluent in German, Russian, Latvian, and English; he said English was the most difficult of the languages he learned. Throughout his life, he had an accent that intrigued the ladies in particular. In 1955, John met a young lady from Topeka named Sally Jo Giffen on a blind date. According to the story, Sally was told by a mutual friend that John was a Latvian prince and that convinced her that he was worthy of consideration. They were married in 1956. Sally continued to work as a dance instructor and John supplemented with part-time work as a short-order cook; he was known to make a mean fried brain sandwich. While at Kansas City, the young couple had their first child, John Edward.

After graduation in 1958, John was accepted for a rotating internship at the Portland Osteopathic Hospital in Portland, Oregon. He and Sally were both enamored with Portland and its beautiful mountains, trees, and rivers, which were a far cry from the flat Kansas countryside and very similar to what John had left behind in Latvia. During the year that John served his internship, the hospital was relocated to a new site and renamed Eastmoreland

General Hospital. Sally was expecting their second child, Dana Christine, at the time, and he used to bring the steaks he was paid to take an overnight call at the hospital home to his expectant wife.

After careful consideration, John decided to locate his practice in Oak Grove, Oregon, a small suburb of Portland. He and a dentist, Elton Storment, DMD, decided to join forces and build a clinic building that is still here to this day. He equipped the clinic with the latest technology, including a sophisticated X-ray room that allowed him to take routine films and even fluoroscopy.

From the outset the practice was a great success. John's charismatic, caring personality and meticulous attention to detail allowed him to develop a following of loyal patients that stayed with him throughout his career. In addition to his practice, he performed free physicals for young athletes, was the team physician for the Milwaukie High School football team and other sports teams, and volunteered his time at the Outside In Clinic in Portland.

He was a loyal supporter of Eastmoreland Hospital and when it came time to increase the capacity of the hospital to one hundred beds, he contributed $5,000 to the building campaign. In the mornings, he would go to the hospital to attend patients admitted to his service. At noon, he would make rounds in nursing homes, and in the evening, he would make house calls. It was not unusual for him to meet patients at all hours in his office or weekends to attend to their emergencies. It was during these early years that daughter Elizabeth Lee was born.

In addition to his demanding practice, he also was an active member of the Elks Club, MAC (Multnomah Athletic Club), and Eastside Racquet Club where he beat his junior partner in racquetball on a regular basis. John always made time for his family, whether it was playing soccer or volleyball in the neighborhood; teaching them to plant and grow a garden; playing chess, backgammon or other games; traveling on vacation; or conversing around the dinner table.

According to his daughter, outside his practice and family, her dad loved the outdoors and enjoyed hunting, fishing, water skiing, travel, and horticulture. His son recalls many instances hunting or fishing with his dad when it was unbearably cold. He also recalled his dad coming home after hunting or fishing, covered with mud or fish guts, and going out to a fancy restaurant or party in the evening.

At the family residence, he would propagate plants such as rhododendrons, and grow a huge garden. He later developed an interest in viniculture that would endure for the rest of his life. To expand his knowledge of the subject, he attended viniculture courses at the University of California Davis. After those classes and classes at the Bert Harris School of Wine Tasting, he began the search for a location where he could raise his own grapes.

He found an ideal location in Dundee, Oregon, and there he planted a 25-acre vineyard of Pinot Noir, Chardonnay, Riesling, Cabernet, and Merlot grapes. Perhaps he liked the Dundee area because it reminded him of the area where he grew up in Latvia.

At the time, the wine industry in Oregon was just getting started. John helped to found the Oregon Chapter of the Knights of the Vine to promote the industry, and was the first grand commander. After his death, grapes grown in this vineyard won an international prize for excellence.

He was involved in medical politics as the president of the Oregon Osteopathic Association and later was one of the two representatives on the Oregon Board of Medical Examiners, serving for eight years, including one year as chairman of the board. He served the osteopathic community in many capacities, including Chief of Staff at Eastmoreland Hospital and president of the Oregon Osteopathic Association.

According to his daughter, her father felt that his greatest achievement was serving as chairman of the Oregon Board of Medical Examiners. His greatest disappointment was the gradual loss of individual control that was being experienced by the medical profession as a whole. To those who were his patients and friends, his loyalty, sense of humor, and intelligence were his greatest attributes. He was passionate about life and showed great appreciation for life's simple pleasures.

Dale Browning, DO 1930 –

In the process of learning more about the history of the osteopathic profession in Oregon, I have been attempting to reach the retired DOs who live in our area. Many of these men were instrumental in my training as an intern at Eastmoreland Hospital. Dr. Dale Browning is one such physician.

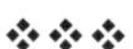

Browning first became interested in the osteopathic profession through the influence of his uncle Floyd Logue, DO, who practiced in The Dalles before the 1940s. Married to his wife Nevelle right out of high school, Browning received his undergraduate degree from the University of Portland on a four-year football scholarship. He was accepted at the Kirksville College of Osteopathy in 1951, and after completing his studies there, he returned to Portland for a rotating internship at Portland Osteopathic Hospital from 1955 to 1956.

After working for a brief period of time with other DOs, he went out on his own, establishing his practice on Division Street near Gresham. At the time, he was the only doctor in the area, and the closest hospital was the old Adventist hospital.

From the day he opened his office, he was busy from morning to night, seeing everything from obstetrics to emergencies. Browning *was* the emergency room in the area for several years.

Throughout his career he continued to refer to and support Portland Osteopathic Hospital and then Eastmoreland Hospital. Browning explained that supporting the osteopathic hospital allowed DO specialists to come to the area to practice, even though it was often inconvenient for him to travel so far to the hospital.

Because of his interest in sports, he naturally gravitated to sports medicine. For many years he was the team doctor for the David Douglas School District and later for Mount Hood Community College, all while attending to his huge practice. Browning also served as the president of the Oregon Osteopathic Association, chief of staff at Eastmoreland Hospital, and was a board member and trustee of that hospital for several years.

He was later joined in his practice by Francis Kai, DO, and another GP. Together they served their community in many capacities. They personally supervised and mentored many osteopathic students and interns in their clinic. They also provided free sports physicals for countless young athletes, and Browning attended every game of David Douglas High School for twenty-three years.

There are many DOs like Browning who serve the profession and their communities with great dedication and distinction. They go about their tasks quietly and without fanfare, yet what a contribution they make.

Robert Butler, DO 1925 –

In October of 2008 and in July of 2014, I had the privilege of interviewing Robert Butler, DO, another of the retirees who still lives in the area and was willing to discuss his career and the history of the osteopathic profession in Oregon. He had a profound impact as a board certified anesthesiologist, educator, and mentor to osteopathic physicians throughout Oregon.

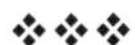

Butler was born in Oak Park, Illinois, a suburb of Chicago. His father, Samuel Butler, was a sales representative for a clothing manufacturer in Bedford, Massachusetts, and his mother, the former Leona Jaminy, was the concert pianist for the Detroit symphony. Butler, the youngest of six children, was the only child to pursue a medical career—and the only child who never learned to play the piano.

Butler's entire educational career was pursued in the Chicago area. He attended elementary and high school in Oak Park; in high school, he played football and proved to be an exceptional speed skater. He was a voracious reader with much of his free time spent in that pursuit. In 1944, he graduated from high school and enrolled as a premed in Roosevelt College, graduating in 1947. During the war years (1941–1945), accelerated higher education was the norm and three years of high school was the standard.

He determined early on that medicine was to be his career. He studied the various medical philosophies, and he decided the osteopathic concept of incorporating osteopathic manipulation into traditional medicine was the best method for treating the whole person rather than the disease. He was accepted at the Chicago College of Osteopathic Medicine in 1947. While attending the school, he supported himself financially by working as a lab tech, an orderly, and at other jobs at the hospital that was part of the Chicago school. He also donated blood every six weeks at the local hospitals for $35 a pint.

At the time, the osteopathic physicians in Illinois were not allowed to admit or manage patients at the local MD facilities, nor were they allowed to prescribe medication or perform major surgery. This was circumvented by courageous DOs who returned to medical school and received MD degrees. W. Don Kraske was one such DO/MD, and it was under his license that the DO residents and students were trained and treated patients at the Hyde Park campus.

In his junior year, Butler met Mary Laug, a nursing student at Wheaton College, and they married when Butler graduated in 1952. After the wedding, Butler returned to Chicago Osteopathic Hospital (COH) to serve a one-year internship followed by a residency in anesthesiology at the same facility. While Butler served his residency at COH, his wife Mary was employed at the hospital as an RN.

While in Chicago, he became acquainted with George Larson II, DO, and after completing his training, the Butlers moved to Eugene in 1953. Butler worked at the DO hospital there and part time at another DO hospital in Albany. Surgical and other DO specialists would come from Portland to assist with the patients admitted to the Albany hospital, but there was not enough work to support his family in Eugene and Albany.

In 1958, Butler and his family relocated to Portland, and resided in the area close to Eastmoreland Hospital for the next thirty-five years. In partnership with Burnham Brooke, DO, Butler provided anesthesia services for that busy surgical service. When it came time to relocate the Portland Osteopathic Hospital, Butler assisted in the development of a department of anesthesia at the new facility on Steele Street. Like so many of the DOs at the time, he actively assisted in the construction of the building and was instrumental in developing the plumbing for the oxygen system and nitrous oxide system of the hospital. From that time until his ultimate retirement, he, Brooks, and various other DO anesthesiologists provided that service twenty-four hours a day, seven days a week.

During his years as an anesthesiologist, he provided training to countless medical students, interns, and residents, never stinting of his time or patience. Perhaps what was most characteristic of this man was his calm demeanor and integrity.

Unbeknownst to many, Butler, a devout Christian, gave time to mission work as well. He started with the World Medical Mission program, providing furlough relief to other doctors who were working in various countries. After his retirement at age sixty-five, he agreed to found a full-fledged anesthesia training program in Kijabe, Kenya, a town located one and a half hours from Nairobi. Along with Wendell Stephens, MD, former head of the anesthesia department at the University of Oregon Medical School, he developed a curriculum for the training of providers with the equivalent of a fifth-grade education. Over the next eight years, Stephens lectured and Butler taught technique, working long hours in the operating room of that teaching hospital, rarely seeing much of the countryside. As a skilled RN, his wife Mary used her knowledge to teach hygiene and child care in the surrounding villages. She pioneered immunization programs that are now used throughout Kenya.

The curriculum at the school is still being used to this day. Butler still has contact with many of his former Kenyan students, and he is confident that they continue to practice safe and competent anesthesia.

As a very busy anesthesiologist, Butler had very little spare time, and, because of the heavy surgical schedule, he was only able to take a week of vacation at a time. His only outside activities were skiing and camping. Despite this, he and Mary raised a fine family of three boys and one daughter. It is clear that the Butlers are a wonderful husband-and-wife team who are an inspiration to those who follow.

His advice to young people considering a career in osteopathic medicine: There is no more satisfying career.

Charles Carlstrom, DO 1903 – 2003

If you travel east out of Portland heading for the ski areas around Mt. Hood, you will pass through the little town of Sandy, Oregon. Extensive forests all around provided the timber that made the place a logging/timber town. It was the perfect location for a DO like Charles "Charley" Carlstrom to set up his practice.

❖❖❖

Carlstom began his life in Hamilton, Montana, where his parents raised their three children. Carlstrom said that an early age he worked in his father's tavern, sweeping floors and polishing glasses. The pay was sixty-five cents a day, a princely sum at the time, making him the "richest kid in the high school" in Hamilton.

After graduating from high school, he worked various jobs until he had accumulated enough money to enroll at Oregon State University in 1929. He joined ROTC to help defray the costs of his education. During his college years, he contracted a severe case of pneumonia that required a long hospitalization and the expense made further education at the time out of the question. Because he had a commission in the army, he became a full-time commissioned officer and served in the army until he was able to resume his college education.

His brother, who had graduated from the Kirksville College of Osteopathic Medicine, urged Carlstrom to apply to the same school.

He was accepted, and he completed his studies at Kirksville in 1941, when he was called back to the army for the duration of WWII. On the day of his graduation from Kirksville, he also married the love of his life, Arrah Young, a Kirksville girl. He had to sell one of his medical books in order to buy a wedding license.

During the war years, he was stationed mainly on the West Coast, including Alaska. He was never allowed to practice as a physician because at the time osteopaths were not considered to be "real doctors." Following his discharge from the army as a major, he completed his osteopathic education as an intern at the osteopathic hospital in Los Angeles. He returned to Kirksville after completing his internship, and he joined his brother Grayton Carlstrom in the area of Malden, Missouri. He became disenchanted with the weather and scenery in Missouri and decided to return the Northwest, an area he had come to love. He had made contact with the DOs in the Portland area during the war years, so in 1948, he contacted one of those DOs, Russ Kanega. On Kanega's advice, Carlstrom relocated his practice to Sandy, Oregon.

After an initial struggle to get things started, his practice thrived. He and Arrah lived above his clinic and he was working or on call almost continuously from that day forward. As was typical of DO GPs, Carlstrom was able to treat just about everything that came through the door of his clinic. He made it a career-long commitment to never turn a patient away. His granddaughter says that oftentimes his pay was a flat of berries or some chicken. (Yes, that did happen in those days.)

He made daily house calls and never wavered from his $5 fee in all the years he practiced. His chart notes consisted of a single line on a 4x8 card. He developed a huge practice that occupied his time and energy seven days a week. He became famous locally for the large Cadillac convertibles that he drove to work and to house calls.

To deliver babies and care for his very ill patients, he traveled to Eastmoreland Hospital, a hospital that he and fellow DOs financed and literally helped to build. After making the rounds of his patients, it was not uncommon for him to be home after midnight.

The hospital had interns and medical students in house most of the time. Often one of these students or an intern worked with Carlstom in the office. Not only did Carlstrom care for a large number of patients, but he was instrumental in the education of many of the DOs in the area as well.

One of the characteristics of osteopathic physicians is a commitment to lifelong learning. Carlstrom was certainly no exception; he attended virtually all of the continuing medical education (CME) offered by the hospital and by the state association. In fact, he attended these sessions long after he had officially retired. He attended AOA conventions as well.

Carlstrom was famous as a "high energy" type of person. He made it a practice to exercise every day by swimming nude in the pool at his home. In addition to the demands of his busy practice, he was very interested in painting and sculpture. He attended art classes at Mt. Hood Community College and created sculptures and paintings galore. In his final days, his small apartment at a local assisted living facility was adorned with many of his works.

Carlstrom and his wife Arrah were strong supporters of the community of Sandy, participating in and supporting a variety of community projects. The Carlstroms were also strong supporters of the arts in the area. They enjoyed the opera and symphony concerts and made a striking pair: he with his shock of white hair, and she dressed in the very latest fashions. Occasionally they would travel, usually to an osteopathic convention or to the CME meetings of the OOA, but also to other parts of the world.

Carlstom officially retired in 1982. Soon he reopened an "office" in the kitchen of his lovely home overlooking Mt. Hood. There he continued to see old patients who couldn't seem to live without his attentions. When Arrah died in 1990, he lived in his old place for a few more years, but eventually moved to Avamere Assisted Living in Sandy.

Carlstom died at age ninety-five, but is still very much remembered in Sandy. You can find furniture from his office and his picture on display at the Sandy Historical Museum. What a contribution this fine doctor made to his community and to the osteopathic profession!

Ned Davies, DO 1922 – 2003

One of the benefits of an osteopathic hospital has been an accompanying training program. Oregon was blessed with such an institution: Portland Osteopathic Hospital, later renamed Eastmoreland General Hospital. When the hospital was first formed in 1944, DOs traveled great distances to avail themselves of the benefits of an osteopathic hospital. That training program produced over 280 graduates, many of whom are in practice to this day.

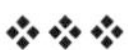

One of the early graduates of the program was Ned Davies, DO, who practiced in Canby, Oregon. After serving in WWII, Davies moved to Chicago to attend college. He earned his way by driving an armored car; the car was also handy for dating his wife-to-be Virginia ("Brownie"). In 1952, he was accepted at the Chicago College of Osteopathic Medicine and graduated in 1956.

The young family then moved to Portland so Davies could serve an internship at Portland Osteopathic Hospital, which he completed in 1957. He chose Oregon because the climate was better suited to his tastes. Like all doctors in the final stages of their training, he began to search for a practice location. He learned of a practice in Canby founded by Milton Mauthe, DO. The practice was later run by Robert Cooney, also a DO. On the first day of his practice, Davies saw only twelve patients, and for a time things were a little slow. According to Davies' son Richard, there were some lean times until the practice began to thrive.

Like so many DOs at the time, Davies plunged into the practice and the community. He assumed the role of team doctor for the high school football program and held that position until Richard took over in the 1970s. He was a scout leader, city physician, and physician advisor for the fire department rescue unit. In fact, he trained the first EMTs to practice in Clackamas County.

During the early years of his practice, he continued to support Portland Osteopathic Hospital, traveling every day to the hospital and back to his office—a long day indeed. Sometime in the 1960s, Davies was approached by the MDs in Canby and invited to join the staff of Oregon City Hospital. He was allowed to join the staff and found that his privileges were even greater than at the osteopathic hospital. He performed appendectomies, gallbladder surgeries, and some gynecological procedures as well. When a second hospital, Willamette Falls Hospital, was built and merged with the old Oregon City Hospital staff, Davies was included on the staff with the same privileges.

His day would begin with hospital rounds at 7:30 a.m. and would end when he closed his office at 7:00 p.m. He was on call seven days a week. (In those days, being "on call" meant you couldn't stray too far from the telephone, because the answering service had to have a number to reach you so you could contact a patient in need. Today's cell phones have definitely freed on-call doctors from being tied to their homes.) Rarely vacationing, Davies' practice was his life.

Davies entered practice at age thirty-six and retired at age sixty-one. He was well known and respected by his colleagues and loved by his patients. A typical small town DO, he put his patients first, yet his sons and daughter thrived. Today one son, Robert Davies, DO, practices in Dallas, Oregon, while the younger son, Richard Davies, DO, has taken over the Canby practice.

Richard Davies, DO 1950 –

The Davies saga continues with Richard. Richard Davies graduated from Chicago College of Osteopathic Medicine in 1975, the youngest graduate that year. He followed his father's footsteps and served a rotating internship at Eastmoreland General Hospital in

1975. Unlike his father, Davies was "booked up" the first day he started practice and has been busy ever since. Like his father, he has been involved in many activities benefiting Canby. He has been physician advisor for the fire department since he arrived in Canby; to this day, he meets weekly with the members of the rescue unit, which now has three ambulances and made 2,500 runs this past year. He is also on call to provide medical advice for the Canby Police Department. In addition, he has been the team physician for the Canby High School football team, and for other sports programs at the school. He does the physicals for the girl's basketball program as well.

Like his father, he tried for a while to support Eastmoreland Hospital, but quickly discovered the travel was too burdensome. He has been an active staff member at Willamette Falls Hospital, serving at one time or another on practically every hospital committee and as chief of staff. He served on the board of directors, and became chairman of the board in 2008.

Davies began his day at 6:30 a.m. by making hospital rounds; he would then head to the office, where he tried to finish by 5:30 p.m. While Davies' father was in practice, the two Davies shared on-call duties; upon his father's retirement, Davies shared on-call duties with two MDs who practiced in nearby Molalla. Davies recently retired after forty years in practice, but he continues to act as physician advisor to the Canby fire department and rescue unit.

Davies has been married to his wife Linda for nearly forty-four years. They have two daughters: Kristin, a charge nurse in the neonatal intensive care unit at the Oregon Health & Science University Hospital, and Beth, curriculum director at Bellevue School District in Bellevue, Washington.

When Richard Davies was asked what was the most challenging thing he faced in practice, he replied that in a town like Canby, where the folks knew him as a little kid and as a cub scout, it was hard to convince some folks that he was an actual doctor now.

His greatest satisfaction has been the success his daughters have achieved. His greatest personal achievement was to be named chairman of the board at Willamette Falls Hospital.

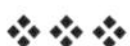

When one contemplates the commitment and energy required to practice osteopathic medicine, be involved in community affairs, and still raise a family, the question arises, "How can this be done?" The answer, of course, is in the tremendous support of the spouse. Ned Davies' wife Brownie "had his back"; through good times and bad, she was there doing all the things necessary to enable the doctor to accomplish what he had to do.

The same can be said for Richard's wife Linda. She carried much of the responsibility for raising the children and the myriad other tasks associated with a home. Richard has always made time to be with his family, joining them for supper, and supporting the girls in their activities.

Both Ned and Richard Davies have made important contributions to the well-being of their community, and are DOs that are inspiration to us all.

William Graham, DO 1935 –

The initial part of the history project I undertook consisted of conversations with retired DOs who live close to me. I am personally acquainted with them and have worked with them during my professional life. Dr. William Graham met all these criteria, but far from being retired, he has continued to practice surgery since 1970 and has no plans of stopping any time soon. Graham has had privileges in every hospital in the greater Portland area and has worked in the emergency rooms of hospitals in nearly every part of Oregon. He has a keen sense of humor and an amazing ability to remember names and dates, which makes him a great story teller—an entertaining and interesting interview indeed.

Graham was the son of osteopathic physician Victor Graham, DO (A. T. Still College of Osteopathic Medicine in Kirksville, Missouri, class of 1933). His earliest memories were of his family residing first in the rear of his father's office and later above it. The office was located in River Rouge, a gritty steel town near Detroit, Michigan. Graham's father worked 9 a.m. to noon, 2 to 5 p.m., 7 to 9 p.m., and often overtime to 11 p.m. It was not at all unusual for him to see ninety patients a day. Of course, there were often emergencies and house calls that extended those hours even more. His mother, a Kirksville native, stayed at home caring for the family.

Graham remembered the local public schools he attended with the children of steel mill workers. Graham's aptitude for science and anything mechanical became evident at an early age. He and two friends all aspired to attend Michigan Tech to become engineers. He was accepted there but instead opted for and was accepted to the University of Michigan School of Engineering. It was required of engineering students to attend Saturday morning drawing classes. Outside the classroom a highly complex model of some sort of machine was exhibited. He was staring at the machine when he suddenly realized that he was going to go into medicine instead. He quickly went from "I will never be an engineer" to "I'm going to study medicine."

He applied to two schools: Chicago College of Osteopathic Medicine and A. T. Still College of Osteopathic Medicine in Kirksville, Missouri. At his interview at Chicago he was so put off by the demeanor of the physician who interviewed him (he said he looked like a used car salesman) that he opted for the school in Kirksville. He graduated from Kirksville with honors (1961) and was accepted at Detroit Osteopathic Hospital (DOH) for his internship. Following his internship, he was accepted into a surgery residency at the same hospital and finished his training in 1965. As a bachelor he was entitled to reside at the hospital and did so until his graduation—a rather monastic existence indeed.

He started his career in surgery in the small town Shenango, Pennsylvania, where he was employed by a DO surgeon at a salary of $15,000 a year while his employer made $140,000. This was in contrast to his salary at DOH, which was $250 per month. The agreement was that after several years, he would eventually split the proceeds of the practice fifty/fifty. The entire agreement was sealed with a handshake—nothing written, no lawyers. Graham said he was totally content with this arrangement until his father had a stroke. He was given a leave of absence to return to Detroit and fill in for his father until he could return to work.

It took longer than anticipated for his father to recover, and during that time Graham's brother, Robert Graham, DO, stepped into his father's practice. At this point, Bill Graham had two decisions to make: Should he return to Shanango under his old contract? No. And, should he marry Mary Lynn Chirila and go on a honeymoon while searching for another place to practice? Yes.

Their search took them to Akron, Ohio; East St. Louis, Missouri; Tulsa, Oklahoma; Albuquerque, New Mexico; Las Vegas, Nevada; a convention in San Diego; Pasadena; and finally Portland, Oregon. There he was introduced to Floyd Henry, DO, and his wife Liz. Graham returned to Chicago for another convention where he again spoke with Henry. He was finally persuaded to locate in Portland, thanks to the efforts of Cleon Miller, DO, Robert Rakozy, DO, and Terry Dierdorff, DO. Initially it was to be a six-month trial, but he soon decided to make Portland his home.

On his first case in Portland, Graham treated an obese man with a hideous abscess in the rectal area. Sometime during or immediately after the procedure, Graham lost his wedding band. Despite this, his wife Mary Lynn stayed with him and bore four beautiful daughters: Natalie, Lori, Megan, and Kimberly. Mary Lynn stayed at home managing the household and raising the girls while Graham devoted all his energies to his surgery career.

As with most of the DO specialists, Graham loved to teach. He worked with students, interns, and residents, allowing them to come to his office to see his patients and to scrub and assist on the many surgeries he performed.

As a general surgeon of that time, Graham was trained in a wide variety of procedures that surgical specialists consider their purview today. He was therefore equipped to deal with virtually any emergency that came to the hospital. When Eastmoreland Hospital closed in 2004, he taught students the art of dealing with minor surgery procedures in an office setting. He continued to accept referrals from the primary care doctors in the area, which often required him to travel long distances to hospitals far from his office. He also was on call for surgical emergencies at these hospitals, usually at night and often uncompensated.

As was typical of DOs of his generation, Graham had few outside interests. He did try to play golf once a week and he had a deep and abiding Catholic faith. During his career he served on many of the committees of the hospital, including a term as chief of staff.

As his primary referring doctors begin to retire, he has been able to cut back his on-call duties and he now covers only one hospital emergency room.

Graham has been meticulous about keeping up to date. He subjects himself to the various competency exams even though this is not mandatory. "Any doctor over seventy needs to be watched," he says. Throughout all the years he has been in practice, he has not lost his passion for surgery and the challenges it presents, as well as the joy of interacting with his patients. His greatest disappointments were the loss of Eastmoreland Hospital and the fact that he is facing the "end of the road." His only regret that he didn't spend more time with his children as they were growing up.

His advice to future DOs: 1. Have a receptive mind and commit to a lifetime of learning and study. 2. Develop outside interests and hobbies. 3. Be in love with your spouse and place that relationship above all others. 4. Always keep your sense of humor!

All in all, a remarkable osteopathic physician.

J. Scott Heatherington, DO 1925 – 2000

Probably the most influential Oregon DO of his generation was J. Scott Heatherington. His devotion to the osteopathic profession, his ability to teach, and his wonderful skill as a politician were all remarkable, but what distinguished him most in the minds of those who knew him and worked with him was his wonderful sense of humor. Rarely was he ever in a situation where he couldn't come up with a witty comment that would defuse a tense situation or make a point that otherwise might not have been acceptable.

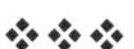

Heatherington was born in the small town of Woodson, Kansas. When Heatherington was nine months old, his father became a minister in the United Brethren Church and was called to his first church in McCracken, Kansas, population 700. There, with his two brothers and older sister, he began his early education. His sense of humor and playful pranks gave him a certain notoriety, which seemed to be the lot of preacher's kids. He was also a redhead.

As is typical of ministers, moving to new churches was a common occurrence and adjusting to new schools was always a challenge. The next church was in Lawrence, Kansas, where Heatherington became interested in music; he played the tuba and later began to sing. While in high school, he also developed an interest in printing and in acting. He was in high school plays and multiple other clubs and societies as well. By his own admission, he did not excel in high school, but chose rather to have fun. Toward the end of his high school career, he began to sing in the church choir, something he enjoyed for many years.

After his graduation from high school, he took biology and twelve hours of college-level classes. To pay expenses, he worked for a small wholesale meat company where he learned how to butcher and prepare meats for the retail market.

One Sunday, a male quartet from York College in Iowa visited his church, and Jerry Dierdorff, the second tenor, talked with him about attending York College. He offered to let Heatherington room with him in a basement apartment with two other students—the rent was seventy-five cents per week plus another seventy-five cents per week for food. Heatherington was the cook.

Regular tuition at the school was $120 per semester, but because his father was a minister, Heatherington's tuition was only $60 per semester. On the first day of registration, he met Gerry Greene, who was also a freshman at York. Heatherington was active in college sports, playing tennis and football. He also was accepted into the male quartet that traveled throughout the Midwest representing the college.

While in college, Heatherington began to consider career choices. The brother of his roommate was an osteopathic physician in Michigan, and it was through this influence that Heatherington began to seriously consider that path as a career. In his third year, he applied to A. T. Still College of Osteopathic Medicine in Des Moines, Iowa, and was advised that he needed to take more premed classes to be eligible. He enrolled in August 1941; not long after he started his medical education, the United States entered WWII. A draft of all young men of certain ages was instituted, but students who were in medical school were exempted if their grades were good. The school instituted an accelerated program where classes were year-round, with a more rigorous and demanding curriculum. His roommate Jerry Dierdorff had gotten married, so Heatherington proposed to Gerry over the phone but Gerry said that he would have to do it in person. So he borrowed a car. Her answer: "Yes! When?" They married in January 1942.

While at school, Heatherington had various jobs, waiting tables at a nightclub and later driving a cab at night. Gerry went to work for an insurance company. In October 1943, his senior year, Gerry gave birth to their first son, Jeff. At the time, it was customary for women to remain in the hospital for ten days, then be in bed rest at home for another seven days. Because Heatherington was a student doctor, they would be allowed to come home after seven days. The ride home was supposed to be in an ambulance, but they couldn't afford that, so some fellow students found a hearse they could use. As they drove down the street, Gerry waved from the windows of the hearse, watching the expressions on the faces of the onlookers.

Heatherington interned at Detroit Osteopathic Hospital. Because of the trying circumstances, he and Gerry reluctantly decided that it would be best for young Jeff to stay with Gerry's parents while he completed his internship. Gerry was able to find work at Chrysler Corporation. After he completed his internship, the young couple was reunited with their son Jeff, and they began the search for a practice location.

After a brief search of possible locations, the family headed west. Jerry Dierdorff was now established in Medford, Oregon, so they began a search for locations in Oregon, and finally chose Medford. Heatherington first had to go to Portland for interviews and examinations with the Oregon Board of Medical Examiners, and he was granted his license on December 7, 1945.

The family had no place to live in Medford, so Heatherington lived for a time with Dierdorff while Gerry and Jeff stayed with a sister in Tulare, California. Heatherington practiced in Medford for twelve years. During that time, two more sons, Doug and Marc, were added to the family.

The osteopathic hospital in Medford at the time was a residence; the obstetrics department was on the third floor of the hospital with no elevator. Heatherington's practice in Medford included delivering babies, covering the ER on a schedule, seeing patients in his office, and making house calls on a regular basis, in addition to doing all of his own surgeries. He was also active in civic affairs, including Salvation Army Board of Trustees, Rotary Club Board of Trustees, Board of Trustees of the Methodist Church, Toastmasters, and the country club. In 1950, he served as president of the Southern Oregon Osteopathic Society.

It was during this time that he met E. L. Burnham, DO, of Gladstone, Oregon. They became good friends and decided to build a new building in Gladstone, where they practiced as medical partners for nineteen years. By then, Heatherington's family had moved to West Linn, Oregon, and the boys were grown.

After arriving in the Gladstone area, Heatherington immediately became involved in local politics. He was a member of the board of directors of the Tri-Cities Chamber of Commerce, board member and president of the Oregon City Rotary Club, president of the Clackamas Knife and Fork Club, president of the Oregon

Osteopathic Association, and member of the House of Delegates of the American Osteopathic Association (AOA).

As a delegate from Oregon to the AOA, he became deeply involved in the national politics of the AOA, and served as its president from 1969 to 1970. In addition to this organization, Heatherington was also a lifelong member of the American Academy of Osteopathic Medicine, serving as its president 1979–1980 and 1991–1992.

After completing his tenure as president of the AOA in 1970, Heatherington was invited to Tulsa, Oklahoma, to serve as dean of the new osteopathic medical school there. He then took a position as director of medical education at Tulsa Osteopathic Hospital.

After five years in Oklahoma, it was time to return to Oregon. There he rejoined Burnham, his old partner, and the two practiced together in Gladstone until Heatherington took the position as director of the department of osteopathic medicine at Eastmoreland Hospital. When Eastmoreland Hospital was sold, Heatherington was called upon to chair the Northwest Osteopathic Medical Foundation, the foundation formed from the funds generated by the sale. As chair, he was instrumental in writing the bylaws of the new organization and in hiring the executive secretary of that organization, David Rianda. This foundation continues to support the osteopathic profession through student scholarships and other activities.

For most of his career, Heatherington continued to practice with Burnham, his long-time partner. Burnham was a strong supporter of Heatherington and would cover for him when Heatherington was on his many trips tending to AOA business. Later the two were joined for a time by Jerry King, DO, and then by Terry Connor, DO, who later took over the practice. Both of the younger doctors were also very skilled as GPs and in the art of osteopathic manipulation therapy.

Heatherington remained on the staff of Eastmoreland General Hospital until he "retired." Like so many other doctors who were on the hospital staff, he served on many of the standing committees of the hospital, and in 1980 he founded the department of osteopathic medicine at the hospital.

Heatherington "retired" repeatedly, but he returned to the hospital several times, each time in a different role. His last role was with the osteopathic manipulation therapy department where he treated patients and helped to train a succession of osteopathic physicians, many of whom are still in practice.

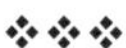

Heatherington was the recipient of many awards over his career. The Northwest Osteopathic Medical Foundation honored him in Oregon as GP of the Year in 1974, and with the Lifetime Achievement Award in 1996. He was honored to be the eighteenth Thomas Northrup Lecturer of the American Osteopathic Association in 1990, and the Scott Memorial Lecturer at the Kirksville College of Osteopathic Medicine in 1991. In 1998, he was awarded the A. T. Still Medallion of Honor by the Academy of Osteopathic Medicine. As a strong proponent of the Jones Counterstrain Method, he was often called upon to assist in the education of osteopathic medical students in Pomona, California. Today, the OMT department at COMP-Northwest is named after him.

After a long and painful battle with cancer, Heatherington died in December of 2000. He is fondly remembered by his students, his patients, and all the organizations that benefited by his participation.

Jeff Heatherington 1943 –

Over the years, the Oregon Osteopathic Association (OOA) has been fortunate in having a succession of executive directors who have been particularly effective in representing the profession in the halls of the state legislature. Despite being in full-time medical practice, these directors and like-minded DOs took the time to be in Salem looking out for the interests of the profession. This is a demanding and often thankless task, which has become more complex and time-consuming than ever before. In 1978, the executive director at the time, Frank Trostel, DO, was instrumental in hiring Jeff Heatherington, a young man uniquely qualified to be the profession's first non-DO executive director.

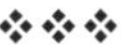

Heatherington was born on October 13, 1943, in Des Moines, Iowa, where his father Scott was attending osteopathic medical school. After his father's graduation, the young family spent a year in Flint, Michigan, where Scott did his internship. At the urging of a fellow student, Jerry Dierdorff, the Heatheringtons moved to Medford, Oregon. At an early age, Heatherington recalls his father's involvement in his practice, in the politics of the hospital, and in community affairs. Scott Heatherington later located his practice to Gladstone, Oregon. The family resided in West Linn, Oregon, where Heatherington and his brothers Marc and Doug attended high school. Heatherington was involved in music, including voice and piano. In his senior year, he became involved in virtually every social activity possible at the school.

When he graduated in 1961, it was understood that Heatherington was destined to follow in his father's footsteps and become a DO. His original plan was to attend Oregon State University (OSU) where most of his friends were headed, but when his father read in Playboy Magazine that OSU was one of the country's top-ten party schools, he strongly encouraged Heatherington to make a more suitable choice. So Heatherington enrolled at Willamette University as a premed student and soon discovered that his interest in premed science topics was marginal at best. In his sophomore year, he changed his major to political science, his lifelong passion. In addition to his studies, he acted as a swim instructor for handicapped children and as a volunteer at the local YMCA. In his junior year, he started a new chapter of the Delta Tau Delta fraternity, which he has served ever since. He was also a Glee Club leader and a volunteer in the chaplain's office.

After graduation from Willamette in 1965, Heatherington served the YMCA in many capacities and locations. After serving in Pasco,

Washington, Heatherington returned to West Linn, Oregon, where he served as director of admissions. He then went to San Diego, where he pioneered the Big Brother program that paired disadvantaged boys with mentors. After this, he returned to Portland to work as business director of the Westminister Presbyterian Church.

To become better equipped as a business director, he took courses in accounting, completing a two-year curriculum in those topics at Portland State University. During this period, he found the time to adopt a boy through the Big Brother program. Today, he proudly displays photos of his grandchildren in his office.

After his time at the church, he took a position as financial director of the Republican Party where he participated in fundraising and became familiar with the art of lobbying.

To relax, he began to take flying lessons, and it was as a member of the flying club that he became acquainted with Frank Trostel, DO. Trostel had realized that his many responsibilities as executive director were interfering too much with his personal life, so he approached Heatherington and broached the idea of Heatherington becoming executive director of the Oregon Osteopathic Association (OOA). The OOA Board agreed and Heatherington was offered the job, which he accepted in January 1978. He hit the deck running, and with all his energy and experience, he began to tackle some of the issues that had plagued the DOs in Oregon.

The state legislature was in session at the time and with the support of the OOA Board, Heatherington introduced a bill that would require Oregon Health & Science University (OHSU) to recognize osteopathic training as a prerequisite for acceptance into their training programs. Despite fierce opposition by the university and the Oregon Medical Association (OMA), the bill passed and was signed into law. In 1981, with the OOA Board's approval and support, Heatherington introduced a bill requiring insurance companies involved in workman's compensation coverage to accept and reimburse osteopathic care in the office setting. This also passed. Passage of these bills required ceaseless effort by Heatherington and dedicated DO physicians. It was not easy.

In 1987, a malpractice crisis with major implications occurred in Oregon when osteopathic specialists and primary care physicians suddenly could not obtain malpractice insurance. The OMA was approached and agreed to underwrite these doctors with the requirement that they become members of the OMA. This mandatory membership requirement did not sit well with the DO community, so Heatherington was instructed to introduce a bill nullifying this requirement. It was a brawl in the legislature, but when the dust settled, the bill eventually passed. Sadly, the intent of the bill was trumped by a federal law that superseded the state law.

The battles never ceased. In 1985, on behalf of Osteopathic Physicians and Surgeons of Oregon (OPSO), Heatherington introduced a bill requiring insurance companies to equally reimburse all Oregon hospitals with training programs. There was heavy opposition, but eventually the bill passed.

In the early 1990s, hospitals began to discriminate against osteopathic physicians in new ways, this time stating only doctors trained in a residency program approved by the American Medical Association (AMA) could be given staff appointments. This sort of discrimination persisted for several years. In 1995, with Heatherington's urging and the support of dedicated osteopathic physicians, the legislature stepped in, stating that any healthcare organization that credentialed physicians must give privileges to all qualified applicants.

In 1991, sunset rules went into effect, including those that governed the Medical Board. Heatherington urged a friendly senator to attach a rider to the enabling bill that changed the status of the DO alternate member on the Board to full membership. How this passed the scrutiny of the AMA lobbyists is still a bit of a mystery. Perhaps Heatherington will confide some day.

As if Heatherington didn't already have enough irons in the fire, he was instrumental in forming FamilyCare, a nonprofit health management organization (HMO) dedicated to the care of Oregon Medicaid patients. Under his leadership and the very able advice of the HMO board members, this became a highly successful enterprise serving over 60,000 clients. From its humble beginnings in April 1985, it is very close now to becoming the second largest Medicaid HMO in Oregon. In the formative years of FamilyCare, Heatherington took no salary. Heatherington very ably wore two hats: executive director of OPSO and CEO of FamilyCare. FamilyCare has contributed over $3 million to OPSO and other osteopathic causes.

Heatherington states that his greatest achievements include his lobbying efforts on behalf of the profession, the development of FamilyCare Inc., raising a fine son and now grandchildren, support of the YMCA and its programs, and being active in the Delta Tau Delta fraternity over the years.

At the dedication of COMP-Northwest, Heatherington spoke for the first time about his involvement in the creation of the school. He had had a conversation with Larry Mullins, CEO of Samaritan Hospital Group in Lebanon, Oregon. Mullins was so intrigued that he invited the administration of the College of Osteopathic Medicine in Pomona (COMP) to visit Lebanon. After considerable prodding by Heatherington, the Pomona folks came to Lebanon and were so impressed that they decided to locate the school there. Of course, the rest is history.

Although Heatherington is no longer executive director of OPSO, he often collaborates with the new executive director, David Walls. The osteopathic profession was indeed blessed to have this man, a strong advocate who was very instrumental in creating the professional climate that exists today for DOs in Oregon.

Floyd Henry, DO 1936 – 2001

Until recently, being a general surgeon in a small osteopathic hospital meant that the surgeon was called upon to perform many different types of surgeries. These surgeons were on call a great deal of the time and were also required to train and mentor future osteopathic physicians. One such general surgeon was Dr. Floyd Henry, who was not only very competent in all areas of surgery, but also made himself available by phone for consultations, often interrupting his day to squeeze a patient into his already busy schedule. His wonderful sense of humor and a relaxed style endeared him to those who worked with him and earned him the respect of the entire medical community, DO and MD. He was a raconteur without peer.

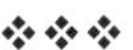

Henry was born in Des Moines, Iowa, into a family of five children, four boys and one girl. His father, an optometrist, and his homemaker mother both had a keen interest in sports, music, and education. As a result, Henry was active in football, baseball, boxing, and piano. From an all-boy Catholic high school, Henry went straight to the all-men's college of St. Ambrose in Davenport, Iowa. In high school, Henry had excelled in boxing and even won a Golden Gloves award. He went on to box for his college team, and also professionally as "Kid Henry" to earn extra money. During college, he began to date Liz Alger, a girl he met at a "mixer" where girls from the all-girl high school met the boys from the all-boy high school.

Initially, Henry's intention was to follow in his father's footsteps and become an optometrist. This all changed when he injured his back boxing and visited the family physician Dr. Barquist, a DO. Barquist inquired as to Henry's future plans, and on a prescription pad jotted the name of the A. T. Still College of Osteopathic Medicine in Des Moines, suggesting that Henry pay them a visit. After a visit to the college, Henry changed his plans and decided to enroll in 1957. Between his second and third year at Des Moines, he married Liz, who was now working as an airline stewardess for TWA Airlines. He graduated in 1961; after a conversation with Milton Snow, another student at Des Moines, he applied for an internship at Portland Osteopathic Hospital in Portland, Oregon. To Henry, the primary attractions of the Northwest were all the opportunities for fishing, hunting, and skiing the area afforded.

Henry met Dr. Richard Scanlon, a general surgeon, during his internship, and soon it became evident that surgery was to be his life's work. After completing his internship, he became a surgery preceptor under Scanlon. A few months later, Scanlon was tragically killed in a car crash, forcing the young couple and their young daughter Suzie to move to Saginaw, Michigan, to continue Henry's preceptorship under Dr. Robert Ferris, DO. They arrived in Saginaw after a very difficult midwinter trip, and Henry immediately embarked on his new responsibilities. As the chief resident, he discovered that he was being paid less than the interns, and he had not had a vacation while at Portland Osteopathic in over two years. Ferris said that this was because Henry had never asked. The work was grueling and the hours were long, but there is no question Henry had a great residency.

There was never any question as to where he would locate. As soon as he could, he returned to Portland where he was royally welcomed. From 1965 to 1970, he worked very hard, often spending the night in the doctor's lounge after a long surgery. Three hours of sleep a night were not unusual, and it was not unheard of for him to have fifteen surgery cases in one day. In addition, he conducted his office practice, consulted, and performed minor procedures, usually with a student or intern accompanying him. He also served as chief of surgery for many years.

During this time, the Henrys adopted a son, Floyd Jr., and a daughter, Katie. Finally, he and Liz had a heart-to-heart discussion—Liz told him he needed to work even harder so that there would be a nice nest egg for her next husband when he died from overwork. And so in 1970, he took a partner, William Graham, DO. Between the two, the hospital had excellent general surgery coverage, and Henry had a little more time to pursue his many outside interests.

During his thirty years in practice, Henry held many offices on the hospital staff, including chief of staff. He was also active in the state osteopathic organization (OOA). He was a wonderful and highly coveted teacher; there was rarely a time when he didn't have a student, intern, or resident working with him. When

Eastmoreland Hospital was sold in 1989, a foundation was formed from the proceeds of the sale. Henry was a founding member of the Northwest Osteopathic Medical Foundation and received its highest award for his service in 2000.

His other interests included trap shooting, golf, and hunting. As his wife Liz would say, whatever he did he did to the best of his ability. That way there were never any regrets about not trying hard enough. He loved a good party, and often his piano playing and stories were the life of the party.

On December of 1995, Henry retired and was able to enjoy retired life, including taking up painting. However, only six months after retirement, he had an abdominal aneurism repair. After the surgery his health quickly began to deteriorate, and a rapid-growing lung cancer led to his untimely demise in 2001.

According to Liz, his greatest achievement was living life to the fullest and caring for people as a surgeon. His greatest regrets were that he didn't spend more time with his family and that he was never able to stop smoking. To this day, stories about this man abound; he had a profound impact on so many osteopathic physicians and their patients. We miss him.

Allan Page Howells, DO 1882 – 1964

In early 1908, the State of Oregon licensed the first group of DOs to practice in the state. Sixty-seven of the original seventy-one applicants were licensed; we have their names but little information as to where and how they spent their careers. On April 21, 2014, it was my privilege to interview Marceil Howells, the widow of one of the earliest DOs to practice in the state, who offered us the first glimpse of DOs who practiced in Oregon in the years following 1908. Her recollections were so vivid that they will be videotaped and become part of the archive being created at COMP-Northwest in Lebanon.

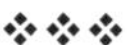

Howells, "A. P." to those who knew him, was born in upstate New York in 1882. At an early age, he was treated by a DO and was so impressed with the result that he decided to make osteopathy his life's work. Prior to attending Colgate University, he was employed by an important book dealer in New York City, Gotham Book Store, and it was during that time that he developed his lifelong passion for study and reading. After graduating from Colgate, he was accepted at the American School of Osteopathy in Kirksville, graduating in 1911. (His diploma can be seen at COMP-Northwest.) His sister, Mary Howells, also graduated from Kirksville at about the same time. The two new DOs located and practiced together in Corvallis, Oregon, starting around 1911. After two years, Howells relocated to Albany, Oregon, and continued in general practice. Mary Howells pursued a career in psychiatry, and after completing studies with Karl Jung in Switzerland, moved her practice to Portland, Oregon.

Howells continued to practice in Albany until the outbreak of WWI. He volunteered to be a physician in the army, but as a DO, he was refused. He was so determined to serve that he applied and was accepted at the Kansas City University of Physicians and Surgeons and received an MD degree in 1919 after the war had ended. (Some of the tuition receipts for various fields of study he completed can be seen at COMP-Northwest; for example, $100 for surgery, and $40 for "colon.") It is not clear whether Howells interrupted his practice while attending medical school, but it is clear that he did return to Albany to practice and continued to do so until his death in 1964.

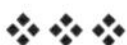

His office was located over a local store in downtown Albany. The office was equipped with a full array of X-ray and laboratory equipment, a surgery, and two rooms for exams and osteopathic treatments. Both his home and office contained volumes that made up a large medical library. He was trained to provide complete care to his patients, including surgery and the treatment of all kinds of emergencies. He read his own X-rays, performed his own blood tests, did his own pathology reports, and performed in-office surgeries such as hysterectomies, gallbladder removals, and T&As (tonsillectomies and adenoidectomies). He also had a "drug room" from which he dispensed various medications. Marceil stated that when she was a girl, Howells was her family's doctor, and when her mother needed a hysterectomy, the procedure was performed right there in Howells' office, with the assistance of a DO associate, Dr. Larry Dennis.

Howells' routine consisted of seeing his patients at his office and making house calls every day in the afternoons or evenings. If an emergency arose, he would often go to the patient. He also had a large *pro bono* practice for families who could not afford medical care. This was especially true during the time of the Great Depression. At that time, office visits were $3, but later increased to $5, with extra charges if X-rays or lab work were required.

His notes consisted of what could be carried on a clipboard and filed in a manila envelope. The records were destroyed shortly after Howells' demise, so we will never know his system exactly. Marceil stated that the confidentiality of the patients' records was a critical trust and the identities of the many *pro bono* patients should never be revealed. At the time of the settlement of Howells' estate, it was suggested that these patients should be billed for services rendered. This was firmly resisted by Marceil, and the records were destroyed.

As was typical throughout the state at the time, DOs were not accepted by the local MDs, and they were often criticized and stymied by various tactics designed to bar them from practice. The most onerous of these practices was the barring of DOs from practicing in the local hospitals. In Albany, Howells and some other DOs formed their own hospital where they were able to admit their patients for surgeries or more intensive care than could be provided in their own offices. As a result of this discrimination, the DOs of the area had strong relationships and provided support to their colleagues. The state association also provided excellent continuing education programs that were well attended by all the area DOs. Howells was often called upon to lecture on various topics, including discussions of what would today be labeled "preventive medicine." He also wrote and published pamphlets for his patients on health topics that he felt were important.

In a profession where constant study was a mandate, Howells stood out. Marceil tells us that he read constantly from medical journals and books. When a patient showed up with an unusual problem, he would determine what the problem was and then search out information on the most up-to-date treatment methods. His wide range of medical studies allowed him to practice a "holistic" type of osteopathic medicine. He often collaborated with his sister Mary and applied the concepts of psychoanalysis to his practice. His breadth of knowledge was often called upon by colleagues when they encountered tough cases.

He was a scholar to the end. On his last day, he saw patients at the office, began to experience chest pains, sat down in his chair at home, and asked his wife to read from a medical journal to help him relax. He refused his injectable medication and died that night.

Marceil also gave us a glimpse of the doctor's personal life. She was his fourth wife, and she was over thirty years his junior. He had two stepchildren from his first wife, four children with his second wife, several stepchildren with his third wife, and three children with Marceil.

Marceil attended high school with one of Howells' sons. The romance between Howells and Marceil consisted of two dates: the first was an afternoon fishing expedition, and the second was a foray to Portland to attend a play. He proposed on the return trip to Albany; Marceil replied that she had to think about it, but this apparently didn't take very long.

Despite their age difference, they had a wonderful marriage. Marceil was an accomplished artist, specializing in the fine arts; she also raised horses, designed and made clothing, farmed, flew airplanes, and raised children. She was also very active in the osteopathic auxiliary and in community affairs.

Howells made it clear that raising the children and running the household were her responsibilities, and that if he wanted her to know something, he would tell her. This situation lasted for a time, but over the years she became his confidante and support in all of his activities. She read his medical journals to better understand what was occurring in a particular case, she often drove the car as he made his house calls, and she occasionally worked in his office as a "fill in."

Howells was a remarkable osteopathic physician who made an important contribution to the health care of the people in and around the city of Albany, and he was married to a remarkable woman who made it possible for him to be the physician he wanted to be.

Lawrence "Larry" Jones, DO 1912 – 1996

In the 1940s, the osteopathic profession began to flourish as never before. During the war years, DOs were called on to fill the void left by MDs that were called into the military. In many small towns in Oregon, a DO was the only doctor in the town. The public quickly recognized that these young doctors knew what they were doing and accepted them wholeheartedly. Dr. Larry Jones practiced in the eastern Oregon town of Ontario for many years.

Jones' story includes the incredible events that led to his discovery of a new osteopathic technique, officially called the *Jones Strain/Counterstrain* technique. This technique is now an important part of the curriculum in every osteopathic medical school in the country, and it is used by physicians and physical therapists around the world.

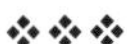

Jones was born and grew up in the city of Spokane, Washington. His father was a civil engineer and his mother was a schoolteacher. His father died when Jones was ten, leaving his mother to support and rear a family of four children on a teacher's salary. It was the time of the Great Depression; to help with family expenses, all of the children had jobs of various kinds. Like so many teenagers of the time, Jones was able to find summer work in the apple orchards of Yakima. While thinning apples, Jones witnessed the effectiveness of osteopathic manipulation. A companion fell from a nearby tree and was unable to walk. Jones's friend called his dad, a DO, who came to the orchard with his table. After one treatment, his companion was able to go back to work. At that moment, Jones decided that he wanted to make osteopathic medicine his career.

After completing the required premed classes, Jones was accepted at the California College of Osteopathic Medicine in Los Angeles, California. He received his DO degree in 1936 at the age of twenty-four, and completed his rotating internship at Los Angeles County Hospital in 1938. His least favorite subject in school was anatomy, yet he later became an expert in the field as his studies of manipulation progressed.

In 1938, he was licensed in Oregon by reciprocity. He had contacted the Oregon State Chamber of Commerce, and with their help, he identified two candidate communities where he might successfully set up a new practice. One was somewhere on the Oregon Coast and the other was Ontario, Oregon. He asked his sister, who lived in Portland, if she had heard of Ontario; she had not, but she suggested instead the town of Huntington. He visited both towns and found that Ontario was a bustling, thriving town while Huntington was a dismal railroad town already in decline. He decided to locate to Ontario and his first office was above a barbershop. Because of his skill at manipulation and medicine, he soon had a thriving practice.

Through a patient who was a schoolteacher, Jones was introduced to Katherine Quast, and soon they were engaged. They married in 1940 after they found a place to rent and were able to purchase an entire houseful of furniture for $150.

During the war years, Jones was called upon to practice as a general practitioner. He covered the emergency room at the local hospital and delivered many babies. Needless to say, he worked very hard and was widely accepted as a physician. He used his skills at manipulation when there was time, but he found that he could not devote the time to it that he would have liked. This all changed in 1945. The MDs returned from the war, and he found he was no longer accepted or wanted at the local hospital. Many of the patients that used his services as a GP continued to follow Jones despite this discrimination. He was allowed to attend the weekly morning continuing medical education (CME) sessions at the local hospital for a while, but when he was no longer invited to these sessions, he stopped attending.

During this time, he attended various osteopathic CME gatherings, including the meetings of the American Academy of Osteopathy (AAO). He worked very hard to stay current.

After WWII, Jones began to devote more and more of his time to manipulation. His skill was widely known and appreciated by his patients in the area. To further his knowledge, he studied anatomy in greater depth and was a regular attendee at the AAO conferences where new ideas were constantly being developed.

In early 1955, a patient was referred to him by a DO practicing in Idaho. The patient's problem was a persistent strain or spasm of the psoas muscle (located along the rim of the pelvis). Despite all efforts, the condition was not responding to methods in use at the time. Jones treated him on six occasions with no success. By this time, the patient stated that if only he could get more than fifteen minutes sleep at a time, he would be happy. Jones decided to experiment. With the patient lying down, Jones moved him gently in various ways until he finally found a position where the patient experienced no pain. He propped the patient with pillows so that the patient could remain in that position while Jones left to see another patient. When Jones returned, the patient was sound asleep. When the patient woke up, he gingerly got up and found that the pain was gone. The patient said, "It's a miracle!" Jones was flabbergasted. (There is a video recording where Jones himself tells this story).

That night Jones paced the floor trying to account for what had happened. Whatever it was, he was going to try it on other patients and see what occurred. What followed was a series of successes as he used this technique on more and more patients in more and more places. Jones's daughter Barbara recalled that at age five, she had injured her neck on a Disneyland ride and had been unable to turn her head since the injury. Jones decided to treat her, and, in spite of her mother's concerns, he placed Barbara on his treatment table and proceeded to move her in various positions. When her head was in a position of extreme extension, she cried out, "That's the goodest of all!" Her neck pain was gone.

Soon he was using his method almost exclusively, rarely using the old high velocity, low amplitude techniques that had been the mainstay of the curriculum at the DO schools. A visit to the Jones home included treatments of guests and family as Jones perfected his method at every opportunity.

This was an important time in the history of the profession. DOs McGoon, Sutherlin, Korr, Denslow, Mitchell, and others were all in their prime, and the literature was replete with their findings and their theories explaining the mechanism of osteopathic manipulation therapy (OMT). They all were well aware that it was very effective, but exactly why it worked was still controversial. Into this group came Jones and his counterstrain technique. In 1966, he published his first paper, entitled "Spontaneous Release by Position," in *The DO* magazine. The concept was not well received by many of his colleagues, but four were so impressed they came to the first class that Jones gave at his home in Ontario. They worked on Jones's patients and had dinner most nights at the Jones residence. These doctors became disciples, returning to their homes and using this amazing technique. Scott Heatherington, DO, was in that first group and was instrumental in teaching students, interns, and residents at Eastmoreland Hospital.

Soon Jones was called upon more and more frequently to give classes on his techniques in other parts of the country and ultimately to DOs and others around the world. Early on he wrote and published a book on the subject, entitled *Jones Strain - Counterstrain*

(Colorado Springs: The American Academy of Osteopathy, 1981), which was translated into many languages.

Despite the proven success of his methods, he was still not widely recognized by the AAO. Jones feared that his method would die with him. In frustration at the lack of acceptance in the academy, he began to present his concepts to other practitioners, including physical therapists. Because of the nature of their practices, physical therapists are able to take more time with their treatments, and the application of counterstrain to their patients was an instant success. Sadly, he was even more vehemently opposed by the AAO because he reached out to the physical therapists.

During this time, his daughter Barbara began to date a young veterinarian from Nampa, Idaho, Dr. Ed Goering. After his daughter's marriage to Goering, Jones and his new son-in-law discovered they shared a lively interest in physiology and biomechanics. Goering injured his back rather severely, and at Barbara's request, Jones made a house call. After just one treatment, Goering was up and working, burning to learn more about this "miraculous" technique. Goering moved his wife and children to Pomona where he enrolled in the College of Osteopathic Medicine of the Pacific (COMP). After receiving his DO degree, the family moved to Portland where he completed a three-year residency in family medicine at Eastmoreland Hospital. Goering now teaches at COMP-Northwest, and continues to give seminars on Counterstrain all over the world.

Despite increasing success, Jones continued to care for his patients and refine his counterstrain technique. He self-published a second version of his book in 1995; like the first, it has been translated into many languages. He continued to teach his method in seminars and increasingly at osteopathic medical schools. The method was especially well received by female students because upper body strength was not an important prerequisite.

❖❖❖

Despite his busy practice, Jones was a member of Toastmasters and later Kiwanis, which he supported throughout his career. These memberships also helped him to hone his public speaking skills. He often paraphrased the biblical saying that a prophet is not loved in his own country. Typical of bright, creative people, he was impatient with the slow acceptance of his method. Finally, in the early 1970s, he became a Fellow in the AAO (FAAO) and began to receive the recognition and respect he so richly deserved. The medical establishment in Ontario never recognized him. You can imagine their surprise when physicians and patients from around the world attended his memorial service in that town.

George Larson II, DO 1918 – 1986

How DOs select the place where they will spend their careers is always interesting and often entertaining. George Larson is certainly no exception.

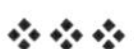

After graduating from the Chicago College of Osteopathic Medicine, Larson hadn't quite made up his mind where to practice. So in 1941, he and his new bride came west to explore an area of the country they had never seen. They made it to the West Coast and were heading south when their car broke down near a little town called Brownsville, Oregon. With his medical background, Larson decided the most knowledgeable person in town would be the local pharmacist. They entered the pharmacy and while waiting, unbeknownst to them, the pharmacist called the town mayor to tell him he had a "live one" in his pharmacy. According to Larson's son George III, in short order his father and his young bride had a practice and a place to live.

For the next ten years, Larson provided the only medical care to the people of the town. As a GP he provided obstetrics, orthopedic, and general practice care.

There were seven saw mills, six churches, four taverns, and a thriving rye grass industry in the area. The demand for lumber during the war years was insatiable and the local mills ran round the clock, so injuries were frequent. (The terminology used by the loggers was a cause for worry and consternation to Larson's new bride. Terms such as "catskinner," "choker setter," and "pond monkey" were all alien to a girl from Chicago.)

There were also fires in the fields of dry grain nearby, creating more hazards. As a result, Larson was on call twenty-four hours a day, seven days a week. He made house calls and was frequently called upon to ride in the ambulance to an injury site where he provided first aid. To facilitate care, he had a siren placed on his car so that he could provide transport for his patients to nearby Albany or Eugene, the closest osteopathic hospitals.

He was also active in community affairs, including acting as fire chief, serving on the school board, and undertaking other civic responsibilities. In those days, pharmaceutical representatives were not permitted to call on DOs, so when the representatives came to town, the local pharmacist would invite them to lunch, where Larson would join them to learn about the latest drugs.

In 1951, Larson decided to change his specialty. For the next two years, he studied obstetrics and gynecology at his alma mater in Chicago. His older brother, Norman, was a professor at the school, and Larson was offered a lucrative position as assistant professor of obstetrics and gynecology. Apparently, Larson's son George III and daughter Karen detested Chicago and were eager to return to the West Coast, so Larson returned, this time to Eugene. There, he joined the staff of Lane Valley Osteopathic Hospital and resumed practice as a GP.

The balance of his career was spent as a GP but his emphasis was obstetrics and gynecology. He was often called to consult on complex cases and performed surgery both at Lane Valley Osteopathic in Medford and at the Albany Osteopathic Hospital.

He continued to pursue his hobbies of boating and auto racing. He was active in Rotary, and held various positions at Lane Valley Hospital. His son George III joined him six months after George III completed his internship in 1971. The two were then joined by Dr. Allen Wallstrom and moved to Springfield in 1980. They continued to support Lane Valley Hospital until it was purchased by Sacred Heart Hospital of Eugene and sold shortly thereafter. Despite severe health problems, Larson continued to practice until his demise in 1986.

Larson was much loved and respected by the people of Brownsville and Eugene. Some of his office equipment can be viewed at the county museum in Brownsville. He was dedicated to his patients and the care of the whole person, a trait shared by many of his fellow DOs. What a legacy and inspiration he is to us all.

Frederick Everett and Hezekiah "Hezzie" Moore, DOs

This biography was written in 2013 by Rhiannon Orizaga, history major, Portland State University.

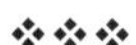

Like many osteopathic physicians in the early 20th century, Frederick Everett and Hezekiah Moore were a married couple who practiced together. They ran a sanitarium from around 1910 to 1925 and were active members in the osteopathic community as well as the Oregon Osteopathic Association (OOA) and the American Osteopathic Association (AOA).

Frederick attended the Northern College of Osteopathy in Minneapolis, the second osteopathic school opened after the American College of Osteopathic Medicine in Kirksville, Missouri. Northern College was established in 1895, so he may have been one of the first osteopaths to graduate from that school. In 1898, he was elected a Trustee of the AOA. He may be related to Dr. A. C. Moore, who founded the Pacific School of Osteopathy in San Francisco the same year, who was also active in the AOA. We do know that Moore had family in California and San Francisco where A. C. Moore practiced.

Hezekiah "Hezzie" Carter Purdom was from Kansas City, and seems to have come from an osteopathic family. Her sister Zudie was a DO who practiced in Kansas City. Hezzie and Zudie both graduated from the American College of Osteopathy; Hezzie probably in 1901. Hezzie was elected Secretary of the Missouri Osteopathic Association in 1902; she was based in Kirksville at that time. Later she was practicing with a Mrs. T. E. Purdom, who may have been either her mother or her aunt. Mrs. Purdom was elected to the AOA in August 1902, the same year that Hezzie was elected as Assistant Secretary.

From November 1901 to May 1902, Frederick was located in Kirksville, possibly taking a post-graduate course. In 1903, he was listed as a graduate of the American School rather than Northern College. Frederick and Hezzie married on June 1, 1903. It is likely that they met in Kirksville at AOA headquarters.

After their marriage, the couple moved to LaGrande, Oregon. On July 17, 1903, they sent a telegram to the National Convention expressing their regrets at being unable to attend, but in 1904, Hezzie attended the National Convention held in St. Louis. Hezzie published an editorial in the *Journal of the American Osteopathic Association* commenting that she would like to see more "practical" papers being presented at future conventions.

The Oregon Board of Medical Examiners was formed in 1907, and Frederick was appointed by Governor Oswald West to be the first osteopathic member of the board. The following year, sixty-seven DOs were granted licenses, including Frederick and Hezzie. In 1911, the couple embarked on a tour of major European and American hospitals to study various treatments and practices. At the same time, Hezzie served as Treasurer of the OOA from 1911–1912.

During their travels, they attended the thirteenth annual meeting of the New York Osteopathic Society, and afterwards visited their families in Missouri and California. In early 1912, they returned to Oregon, where they practiced in an office suite designed to their personal specifications in the newly constructed Selling Building in Portland. (Today the Selling Building is on the National Register of Historic Places).

Frederick was reappointed to Board of Medical Examiners in 1912. He also served as the Chair of the Program Committee of the OOA. Hezzie served as treasurer and later as editor of the OOA newsletter. That year, the OOA extended an invitation to the AOA to have the 1915 annual convention in Portland.

Frederick retired from his position on the Board of Medical Examiners in 1917 and was replaced by Dr. D. D. Young.

Around this time, Frederick became a firm believer in the "milk cure" and presented a paper at the annual OOA meeting entitled "The Milk Cure for Certain Chronic Diseases." The Moores were treating patients with this method while maintaining their office in the Selling Building, and by 1919, a travel diarist referred to Frederick as the "Milk Man" of Portland.

By 1922, they had established the Moore Sanitarium on Hawthorne Street in southeast Portland. Advertisements for the Moore Sanitarium appeared regularly in osteopathic journals with slogans like "How Does Milk Cure?" Milk cures disease simply because it supplies elements required to make new blood in abundance. Combined with osteopathic treatment and rest, wonders can occur in a few weeks. The advertisements focusing on the Milk Cure hint that the Moores were no longer interested in "pure" osteopathy.

The early 1920s were a tumultuous time for osteopathic medicine in Oregon and indeed the entire country. There were conflicts between DOs insisting on treatment using "pure" osteopathy and DOs who began to incorporate alternative methods, such as the Electronic Reactions of Abrams (ERA), into their treatment programs. Frederick was one of many DOs who became interested in the ERA method and combined it with osteopathy in his practice. There is little evidence that Hezzie was in favor of or personally endorsed this method.

Their practice was thriving and some in the osteopathic community respected them, but many in the community were not in favor of ERA and regarded DOs who did use the method with suspicion. Elections in the AOA reflected a conservative trend, and after 1920, neither of the Moores served in any capacity in the AOA or OOA.

At the annual meeting of the AOA in June 16, 1923, Frederick delivered a short address to the seventy-five members who were present. That same year, he attended a ceremonial laying of the cornerstone for the new ERA school in San Francisco. Upon Frederick's return to Oregon, the couple continued to practice together, running their office and the sanitarium. The Moores began to advertise the addition of ERA to their sanitarium practices.

In 1923, the editors of *The Western Osteopath* called for submissions to allow supporters on both sides of the ERA debate to defend their positions. The same year, the Missouri Osteopathic Board passed a resolution that made it clear that osteopathy and ERA were not to be mixed.

In January 1924, Frederick attended Albert Abrams, the founder of the ERA method, as Abrams was dying. After Abrams' death, Frederick spent several weeks in San Francisco, attending Abrams' funeral and spending time at Abrams College. He accepted the post of president of the Abrams School, now named College of Electronic Medicine, in April of 1924. He moved to San Francisco without Hezzie, who stayed in Oregon to close the sanitarium. Information about the Moores after 1924 is scarce.

Their career trajectory is sad and could be a cautionary tale. Abrams' Electronic Reactions were eventually proven to be complete nonsense and are regarded by the profession as part of regrettable era in which quacks successfully preyed upon gullible people. The Moores were not the only DOs or MDs from Oregon to subscribe to Abram's ideas and other strange notions, but as a high-profile osteopathic practitioner, Frederick's involvement in such dubious methods was unfortunate.

Larry Mullins, DHA 1949 –

If you drive to Corvallis, Oregon, and take the Pacific Highway north, you will come to a small side street called Elks Drive. After a short distance on Elks, you come to Samaritan Drive and the entrance to what, at first glance, seems to be a lovely college campus. The many trees obscure the buildings of what is actually the campus of Good Samaritan Regional Medical Center. Everywhere you look, there is evidence of new construction and bustling activity. The main hospital building also serves as the corporate headquarters of Samaritan Health Services and the offices of its dynamic president and CEO, Dr. Larry Mullins. Many of the new buildings have been constructed since he took the post of hospital administrator twenty-three years ago. This is the story of his career and his contribution to the osteopathic profession.

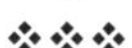

Mullins was born to Richard and Lucille Mullins in the town of Lakewood, Ohio. His early years were spent with his two brothers, David and Lee, and his sister, June, in Ohio, until his father, for health reasons, moved the family to Phoenix, Arizona. Richard found employment as a maintenance engineer in a local nursing facility there, while Lucille worked as an admitting clerk at a local hospital, and later in accounting. Mullins attended Moon Valley High School in Phoenix, graduating in 1968. He was active in football and track, but was still expected to work. One of his first jobs was as a dishwasher at a nursing home, and later he worked as a maintenance man.

The Vietnam War was going on at the time, and the draft of young men was universal. Following his brother's example, Mullins enlisted in the Marines even before he graduated from high school. After his graduation, he was immediately sent to the San Diego training center and later to Camp Pendleton for combat training. By age nineteen, he was already involved in combat missions including beach landings and helicopter insertions; by age twenty, he was a much-decorated veteran. He was rotated back to the United States and spent his last six months at El Toro Air Base in California. During that period, he enrolled in the local community college, beginning a rapid educational ascent to his doctorate in health management years later.

Following his service in the Marines, he married Barbara Hibner, his high school sweetheart. Mullins says that without her loyalty and staunch support, he never would have been able to endure all the hardships and challenges he faced in the war.

After discharge, Mullins enrolled in Glendale Community College in Arizona, and while attending Glendale, had a job as an orderly at a local hospital. His major at the time was history and science with the goal of becoming a teacher, but he changed his field to health care after working in the hospital. He graduated in 1973 and became a licensed registered nurse, then promptly enrolled at Arizona State University.

With his RN degree, Mullins was better able to support himself and his family, first as a floor nurse, and later in the Emergency Department and in various supervisory capacities. This income and the GI Bill enabled him to complete his bachelor of science in health science in 1976, and enroll in a master's program at Northern Arizona University. He obtained his master's degree in education and psychology in 1979.

Not long after graduation, Mullins found a job as an assistant administrator at Valley View General Hospital, an osteopathic hospital and skilled nursing facility near Phoenix. To become an administrator in such a facility, Mullins had to obtain a hospital administration license from the State of Arizona.

The Baptist Hospital chain purchased Valley View, and soon Mullins was leading various projects for the group, including the development of the first private sector helicopter rescue in the state. Over the next twenty years, Mullins steadily advanced up the management chain to senior vice president, with a host of accomplishments, including the construction of new hospital in Glendale.

In 1992, a close friend advised him that the Good Samaritan Hospital in Corvallis, Oregon, was searching for a new administrator. After several interviews, he was offered the job. After discussing the move with his wife and family, he accepted the job and moved his family to Corvallis.

In 2003, Mullins obtained his doctorate in health administration at the Medical College of South Carolina. His dissertation was a study of hospital emergency preparedness, and it is still used as a reference at that school and other colleges.

With the needs of the mid-Willamette Valley foremost, Mullins and his Board of Directors at Good Samaritan Hospital embarked on an ambitious program of modernization and expansion of services. To fulfill the surgery needs of several hundred cardiac patients, the hospital opened a cardiac surgery unit, and a helicopter service was developed to transport these patients from other areas of the valley in emergencies. For patients with kidney challenges, a dialysis unit was created. The emergency room was upgraded to a Level II facility to assure sophisticated emergency care for these and other patients. A neurosurgery department was developed to serve the increased needs of the Emergency Department.

Soon, Samaritan reached out to smaller community hospitals in Lebanon, Lincoln City, Newport, and Albany to form a health care system called Samaritan Health Services. Members of this new health system were able to benefit from all the services offered by the centrally located Corvallis hospital.

At the time Mullins arrived, one urgent task was to recruit more physicians to the area. Mullins instituted a practice development program, which began with two physicians. The practice development program has proven to be widely successful, and now has more than four hundred physicians, physician assistants, and nurse practitioners providing care.

Despite this large group, there was still a shortage of physicians and nurses. In conjunction with the community's Linn Benton Community College, an existing nursing program was expanded, and programs were formed to offer training for laboratory and X-ray technicians. Many of these graduates stayed in the area to be employed by Samaritan Health Services, directly benefitting the organization and community.

In 2006, Samaritan Health Services began to accept third- and fourth-year osteopathic students from the College of Osteopathic Medicine, Pomona (COMP) for clinical rotations. Later, residency programs in family medicine, general surgery, internal medicine, and psychiatry were instituted. More residency programs were added, including orthopedic surgery, pediatrics, and two cardiology fellows. A large percentage of these new doctors are remaining to practice in Oregon, and today there are close to ninety osteopathic residents in various programs with Samaritan Health Services.

In 2007, Mullins attended a meeting where he became acquainted with Jeff Heatherington, chairman of FamilyCare, Inc. In conversation, Mullins mentioned to Heatherington that the health organization had been bequeathed a fifty-acre plot right across the street from the hospital in Lebanon, and the Board was considering a medical school for the site. Heatherington passed the word to the leadership at COMP, and a visit was arranged.

Mullins met Ben Cohen, provost, and Philip Pumerantz, president of Western University of Health Science, at the Hilton Hotel in Corvallis. The three drove in Mullins's pickup to Lebanon to look at the town, the Good Samaritan Hospital, and the site of the proposed osteopathic medical school. Mullins said that the staff at the hospital and the people of Lebanon were very welcoming and convinced the visiting doctors that this would be a wonderful site.

Mullins relates that the negotiations related to the many details of this project took about two years. During that time, he used his persuasive powers to convince the Samaritan Health Services Board of Directors that this project would be a tremendous addition to the town and well worth the financial investment. Construction of the school began in 2009, and the first class began their studies in 2011.

Not long after the school opened, the Oregon Department of Veterans' Affairs agreed to construct a long-term care facility for veterans on the same site. Other projects are moving along as well, including a new convention center, hotel, restaurant, and healing garden. Every new structure reflects Mullins's passion for service to his community.

❖❖❖

Mullins's daughter Jennifer has two sons, Jackson and Garret, and works in the health care fundraising field in Arizona. His son

Robert is now in administration at Samaritan Lebanon Community Hospital, overseeing business development of the campus. Mullins now enjoys travel with his wife, Barbara, and the occasional round of golf.

A host of other projects are on the drawing board for the fifty-acre site on the Samaritan Health Sciences campus in Lebanon, along with projects across Samaritan's service region. The street in front of the new medical school, COMP-Northwest, is named Mullins Drive, a fitting tribute to this remarkable man.

Ira J. Neher, DO 1901 – 1994

In the years following the 1927 legislative action that broadened the scope of practice of the osteopathic profession, DOs were finally allowed to practice in the manner in which they had been trained. DOs could now prescribe medication and perform major surgery, but they still faced formidable challenges. In Oregon, the timber-based economy was in the doldrums and practice opportunities for new DOs were few and far between.

Established DOs were wary of new DOs competing for their patients, and the patients were suspicious of DOs who were prescribing medication and performing major surgery when only a few years before all they could do was "bone cracking." Into this difficult climate came an optimistic and energetic young DO who led the way to a new beginning for the osteopathic profession in Oregon.

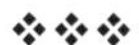

Ira J. Neher was born in October 11, 1901, in a small farming town in North Dakota. Early on the Nehers moved to Wenatchee, Washington. Neher and his brother and sister attended school in Wenatchee, and it was in high school that Neher met his lifetime sweetheart, Lila. Little is known about summer jobs for the children, but it is known that his brother sustained a serious injury in the apple orchards and was attended by the family osteopathic physician located in Wenatchee.

In 1919, Neher was accepted at Willamette University in Salem, Oregon, graduating in 1924. While attending Willamette, his brother-in-law, a student at Los Angeles College of Osteopathic Medicine in Los Angeles, advised him to consider osteopathic medicine. He was accepted at the Los Angeles College in 1923.

He married Lila in 1925. He had to drive his Model T Ford from Los Angeles to Wenatchee in time for the December 28 wedding; considering the roads and the season, it must have been an epic journey.

Following graduation in 1928, he served a one-year rotating internship at The Sanitarium in Arbuckle, California, then trained for an additional six months in surgery and obstetrics at Nugent General Hospital in Centralia, Washington.

In 1930, Neher came to Portland and set up practice with Claude Pengra, DO, the only other "hospital trained" DO in Oregon. Because of his extra training, Neher made an arrangement with Dr. Nicholson, who owned Portland General Hospital in the Sellwood area of Portland. Neher was permitted to perform surgery and deliver babies at that hospital, but was forbidden to sign birth certificates or make progress notes on the patients under his care. This was a business decision on the part of Nicholson, who needed patients to fill the beds of his proprietary hospital. Neher was frequently brought up before the Board of Medical Examiners for practicing medicine without a license, pharmacists often refused to fill his prescriptions, and school nurses would refuse to accept his signature on student health documents. "Detail men" (representatives) of the various drug companies were expressly forbidden to visit DO offices. Only one insurance company, Mutual of Omaha, would cover DOs.

As the years went by, patients became aware of Neher's expertise, his caring attitude, his wonderful sense of humor, and his humble approach to the practice of osteopathic medicine. As WWII approached and more and more business was coming to Portland General, Nicholson made it increasingly difficult for Neher to continue to practice at that hospital. By this time, several other DOs had located in the Portland area, and they were all fed up with the shabby treatment they were receiving at Portland General.

In 1944, Neher and fellow DOs Leonard Purkey, William Hinds, and Joseph Long decided to incorporate a hospital. With the help of physicians, families, and friends, an old building on 616 NW 18th was soon converted into Portland Osteopathic Hospital. Long served as the chairman of the hospital, and the hospital board consisted of Purkey, Hinds, Harold Larson, Carey Martin, George McGovern, and A. B. Reynolds. The new osteopathic hospital thrived.

With Neher as chief of staff and chief of surgery, a number of osteopathic specialists were attracted to this thriving enterprise. As the hospital continued to grow, it became evident that a larger facility was needed. Under Neher's leadership, a new location was found in the Eastmoreland area. In 1974, the hospital was renamed Eastmoreland General Hospital to emphasize the broad capabilities of the new hospital. From 1944 until the hospital finally closed in 2004, students, interns, and residents in family medicine were trained at this facility.

During these years, Lila Neher played an important role, first as nursing supervisor of the Portland Osteopathic Hospital and later as an RN at Eastmoreland Hospital. In addition to his many duties at the hospital, Neher found time to serve on the board of the Oregon Osteopathic Association, including a term as president in 1955. In 1956, Neher became a trustee of the American Osteopathic Association Board of Directors, and he served as a member of the Oregon State Board of Health and Hospital Survey and Construction. In 1967, he received the Distinguished Service award from the Oregon Osteopathic Association.

During these many years of service, the Nehers had two daughters, five grandchildren, and one great-grandson.

Neher's greatest contribution to the osteopathic profession and to the people of Oregon was the leadership he provided in founding the first osteopathic hospital in the state and later to the founding of the Forest Grove Community Hospital.

His sense of humor, kindness, perseverance, and loyalty to the osteopathic profession are examples to all who follow in his footsteps.

Rolland O'Dell, DO 1946 –

On May 3, 2011, I was delighted to interview Rolland O'Dell, the first osteopathic cardiologist in Oregon and probably in the entire Northwest. O'Dell represented a new type of DO, a highly trained osteopathic specialist. Along with other osteopathic specialists he helped to elevate the quality of care at Eastmoreland Hospital in Portland to a new level, providing high quality education to the students, interns, and residents, and superb care to the patients.

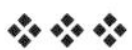

Born and raised in the Portland area, O'Dell attended local schools and took his premed classes at Portland State University. During that time, he encountered a local DO, Robert Rakozy, who discussed with him the possibility of osteopathic medicine. When the time came, O'Dell was accepted at the Kirksville College of Osteopathic Medicine. He graduated in 1972, and was accepted at Tulsa Osteopathic Hospital for his rotating internship. Following his internship, he continued his education as a resident in internal medicine at the same facility. He was accepted at three cardiology fellowship programs after his residency, but he opted for the University of Oklahoma.

After graduating from medical school, he married his wife Diane, also an Oregonian. They met in the romantic setting of zoology class at Portland State. By the end of his cardiology fellowship, the first of three children was in the picture, so early employment was a priority. After turning down several offers in Oklahoma and elsewhere, the young family returned to Portland.

O'Dell applied to Eastmoreland Hospital, where he initially received a chilly reception. Apparently, cardiology coverage was just fine with the general internists already there. Luckily, a cardiac surgeon at Emanuel Hospital needed a cardiologist to consult. To make this happen, O'Dell applied for privileges at Emanuel, and by this time, at least officially, most of the barriers to DOs had been overcome. However, this did not prevent individual MDs from requesting that their patients not be attended by DOs. In his second year, O'Dell was recognized by the house staff as Educator of the Year.

In the second year as a cardiologist assisting the cardiac surgeon, he was joined by Robert Olson, DO, and the two later formed a partnership that served the osteopathic community well.

Like so many other DO specialists, O'Dell devoted a great deal of his time to education. Rarely was he without a student, intern, or resident at his side at the hospital or in his office. He was trained in a rigorous, demanding program, and he tried to use the same standards, giving him the reputation of being a tough but fair mentor. He loved to teach, and was often called upon to educate his fellow DOs, paramedics, and others in cardiology. He had an excellent rapport with his patients, and all those who came to him for care came away with a very strong understanding of their condition and how important it was to take responsibility for their own health.

O'Dell was always readily available to the primary care doctors who relied on him for consultations and advice, (This was one of the characteristics of most of the consultants who worked at Eastmoreland Hospital.) Rather than relying only on a written consultation that could be lost in the sea of paperwork, O'Dell personally contacted the referring physicians and reported his findings and recommendations.

Although O'Dell is now retired, he is still active in education and provides in-depth education in cardiology to the students rotating through the Northwest track of the new A. T. Still School of Osteopathic Medicine in Phoenix, Arizona. Judging by his youthful appearance, O'Dell is practicing what he preaches.

O'Dell states that his greatest satisfaction came from demonstrating, along with other specialists, that it was possible to provide medical care in a small osteopathic hospital that was comparable or superior to other hospitals in the Portland area. His greatest disappointment was when Eastmoreland Hospital was closed so abruptly. His hope is that the new osteopathic medical school in Lebanon will help to maintain the spirit of collaboration and concern for patients that so characterize the osteopathic physician.

Erling J. Oksenholt, DO 1948 –

One of the important factors distinguishing the osteopathic profession has been that so many of these physicians have located in small towns. The impact these doctors have made on their communities has been remarkable. In the town of Lincoln City on the Oregon Coast is such a physician, Dr. Erling J. Oksenholt. Oksenholt has not only made important contributions to the care of the people of Lincoln City but also in many countries around the world.

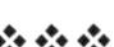

Oksenholt was born into a family of high academic achievement; his father had a PhD in history, was fluent in ten languages, and taught history at a college in Addis Ababa, Ethiopia. His mother was also an educator. Oksenholt and his brother Robert and sister Bertha spent their early years in Ethiopia, learning to speak the language fluently. Academic excellence was expected in the home, and all three children excelled. When Oksenholt was twelve, his parents decided that it would be necessary to move back to the United States in order to further the education of their three children.

In Ethiopia, most of his friends had parents who were medical people, so he and his friends were often found at the local hospitals or clinics, helping to attend to the many poor who were ill or disabled. It was during that time that he decided to become a doctor.

His father took a position as a teacher at a high school in Montana. When it was time for high school, Oksenholt, and later his brother and sister, were sent off to the Mt. Ellis Academy in Bozeman, Montana. Since the school was over a hundred miles away, the children stayed in Bozeman while their parents were in another town. Oksenholt excelled academically, and still found time to be involved school politics. He graduated after three years in 1964.

After high school, Oksenholt attended college at Walla Walla College, an Adventist College in Walla Walla, Washington. There he again excelled. In addition to his studies, he found time to turn out for soccer and work on the school paper in many capacities, including editor. While at college, he met his wife-to-be, Joan Bruer, who was a teaching major from the Seattle area. Until his senior year, he intended to attend an allopathic medical school, but a career advisor mentioned that the Kansas City College of Osteopathic Medicine never had Saturday classes. As a devout Seventh-Day Adventist, observation of the Sabbath (Saturday) was crucial.

In 1968, he married Joan and was accepted into the Kansas City College of Osteopathic Medicine. As always, Oksenholt excelled academically, and also served as the editor of the school newspaper. He was given great latitude in what was included in the paper, and more than once the college president called him on the carpet to explain articles that rankled alumni or faculty. He said that he and the president got to be on a first name basis. While in school he met DOs who would later come to Oregon, including Jay Betts and Jon Nelson.

After graduation, he served his internship in the new osteopathic hospital in Kansas City, and he found he had many wonderful opportunities to learn at this huge new hospital. He was offered several residencies during that year but remained steadfast in his desire to be a primary care physician.

When deciding where to locate in practice, he and his wife had several criteria in mind. They desired a small town with an Adventist presence in the area and potential for growth. After considerable "shopping" for a location, they answered an ad placed by an MD that stated Lincoln City, Oregon, was in need of more doctors. After careful consideration, the fact that there was a brand new, well-equipped hospital led the young family to decide that Lincoln City would be the place.

On arrival, Oksenholt hit the town in a hurry, and soon he was involved in the hospital ER, in clinical practice, and in the training of the local fire and rescue department in the latest techniques. Forty years later, he is still deeply involved in the training and advising of emergency medical technicians (EMTs). Lincoln City is right on the Pacific Ocean, and it was not unusual for fishermen or recreational swimmers to nearly drown in the cold waters. The victims were brought to the nearest hospital for treatment for hypothermia. Oksenholt quickly became the leading expert on the condition in the area. He wrote a chapter on the topic in *Conn's Current Therapy*, a medical reference book. He also wrote numerous journal articles and made presentations around the country. To date, he estimates that he has treated over one hundred victims who would never have survived otherwise.

Oksenholt arises each day at 4:30 a.m., studies for an hour or two, and then walks to the nearby hospital, where he is the ER supervisory physician. He then goes to his clinic where he sees patients until 6 or 7 p.m. He takes one day a week off—the Sabbath.

Early in his career, he became interested in medical missionary work. He began to form teams which initially travelled to the jungles of Brazil, treating—and more importantly, educating—the villagers. He stressed practical treatments; for example, a combo of butter and sulfur for scabies. These simple remedies could easily be taught to the medicine men. Later he and his team returned to Ethiopia, and in 1998, he began a program that has developed into a teaching hospital, several clinics, an orphanage with one hundred children, and a high school with over one thousand students. Many of these programs were the result of Oksenholt's leadership and collaborative skills. He has also led teams to Borneo, Lesotho, New Guinea, Peru, Solomon Islands, Tanzania, Zambia, Rwanda, and Thailand. All of these efforts, and the teams consisting of thirty to forty volunteers, are self-sufficient.

To keep himself up to date medically, Oksenholt has competed for several years in a program sponsored by the Cleveland Clinic called the Smartest Doctor Competition; he recently placed sixth in a group of eight thousand doctors. He has become board certified by the American Academy of Family Practice (and recertified every six years since 1984) and also by the American College of Family Practice, Emergency Medicine, Sports Medicine, and Geriatrics; most recently he is studying for recertification in Geriatric Medicine.

Since starting practice forty years ago, Oksenholt has always had medical students and residents. They come from various schools; most recently from Oregon Health and Science University and beginning in 2014, from COMP-Northwest. His missionary teams often include residents and students, thus providing invaluable exposure to the "real world" for these young people.

Oksenholt and his brother Robert are affiliated with the Samaritan Hospital Group located in Lebanon. Robert, an osteopathic pulmonologist and specialist in intensive care medicine who practices in Albany, suggested the idea of an osteopathic medical school in Oregon to his boss Larry Mullins, CEO of Samaritan Group. Oksenholt also spoke with Jeff Heatherington, chairman of FamilyCare Inc. and former executive secretary of Osteopathic Physicians and Surgeons of Oregon (OPSO) and as a result our new osteopathic school in Lebanon, Oregon, is now in operation.

The Oksenholts have two children, son Erling Jon and daughter Karina Joan, and four grandchildren. In his leisure time, he enjoys ham radio operation and coin collecting.

Oksenholt states that he loves what he does and has no plans to retire. When asked if he used osteopathic manipulative techniques in his practice his answer is yes, once or twice a day. He feels that his osteopathic education prepared him for a career where the patient comes first—the joy is the giving of yourself, not how much you can earn.

David E. Reid, DO 1910 – 1986

The opening of the osteopathic medical school in Lebanon amazed and inspired many Oregon DOs. Most of those osteopathic physicians can well remember opposition, both locally and in the state legislature, from the AMA, the OMA, and other groups, but ultimately, the osteopathic medical school came into being. One of the early DOs who was instrumental in paving the way was David Reid, DO.

❖❖❖

Born March 19, 1910, to David and Gwendolyn Reid, his formative years were spent in Chico, California, where he excelled in athletics and academics. After studying A. T. Still's teachings on the concept of osteopathic medicine, he decided to become an osteopathic physician.

After graduation in premed at Chico State University, he worked a variety of summer jobs, including stringing power lines across the western United States. He was accepted at the Kirksville College of Osteopathic Medicine; to pay his expenses there, he worked as a short-order cook and also took extra classes in anesthesiology. He graduated in 1931, followed by an internship with a married DO couple in Arbuckle, California. After completing his internship, he visited a number of towns in California, Nevada, Idaho, and Oregon, searching for a small town where he could practice. In 1933, he settled on Lebanon, Oregon, a town where the motels didn't have bed bugs and the local MDs were receptive to having another doctor in town.

At the time, there was plenty of work for every doctor. What made Reid stand out was his training in anesthesia. He was immediately allowed to practice in the local hospital and was soon giving anesthesia (mainly ether drip). When the community applied for a Hill Burton grant to build a larger, more modern hospital, Reid had strong support from both the community and his fellow physicians to be on staff at the new facility. Reid was also instrumental in fundraising for the hospital. This acceptance of a DO on the staff an MD hospital was quite unusual at the time.

When Reid arrived, Lebanon was a bustling town with logging, sawmills, and agriculture as the main industries. The timber industry work was sporadic. The saw mills were sometimes closed temporarily because of lack of demand for lumber, or the forests might be closed to logging due to dry weather conditions. This meant workers were often laid off for varying periods of time, and during those down times, it was very difficult for the workers to support their often large families. Reid carried many of these families on his books, accepting barter goods or free labor at his house as payment. During WWII, however, the pace became frantic, with the mills running round the clock seven days a week. The demands on physicians became nearly overwhelming, making it almost impossible to vacation. Often the on-call doctors would be called from church or other activities for emergencies. Reid made house calls practically every day; during a severe flu epidemic, he visited nineteen patients in one day.

Despite the demands of his practice, Reid found the time to be involved in a multitude of community affairs. He belonged to Rotary (secretary/treasurer), acted as chief of staff at the Lebanon Hospital, and was active in the Elks Lodge, the Masons, his church, and on the boards of Lebanon Union High School and Linn County Community College.

While serving on the high school board, there was a discussion regarding whether the school needed a new gym. When Reid opposed the proposal, he was invited by the superintendant to visit the gym. While walking on the floor of the gym, a rotten board gave way under him. The school got the new gym.

One of Reid's passions was Oregon State University sports. He was an honored member of the Beaver Club and had special seats at Gill Coliseum and at Parker Field. In fact his lifelong friend and local pharmacist, Bob Adams and his wife Betty (Adams' Rexall Drug), still have those seats to this day.

Another of Reid's lifelong passions was his love of the circus. According to his daughter, Marsha, as a little boy Reid was quarantined at his home for a time and missed the local circus when it came to town. The circus folks heard that the little boy couldn't attend, so they came to his home and performed in the street outside his house. From then on, he was hooked. When he came to Lebanon, he always took the day off from his office to attend the local circus, and he endeared himself to the circus folks by performing an emergency appendectomy on one of their trick seals. He later became friends with Clyde Beatty, a famed animal trainer, when he sewed up a claw laceration on Beatty's assistant. Reid knew the names and unique makeup of all the registered clowns in the United States, and when they were in town, the performers would come to his home for a party and to perform their acts in his yard. Reid had an extensive collection of circus memorabilia; sadly, the entire collection was lost in a fire not long after his death.

Bob Adams, a local pharmacist and close friend, tells an amusing story about Reid. Shortly after Adams bought the pharmacy in Lebanon, Adams found a note on the prescription counter stating that Reid had been in the pharmacy after hours to pick up some medication needed by a patient. He had a key to the pharmacy which he kept for all the years he was in practice.

For recreation, Reid loved ballroom dancing. While attending a dance, he noticed a young woman, Nell Fisk, a local girl who was the orchestra leader's girlfriend. Despite this, Reid invited her to dance, and later they became permanent ballroom dancing partners. Together they formed a dance club that had functions in and around Lebanon for years to come. They later married, and they had two children, David E. Reid III and Marsha A. Reid (Ms. TygJules SkyWatcher).

At six feet, eleven inches and three hundred pounds, Reid was a commanding presence. People noticed him wherever he went, but he was always described as a gentle giant. Because of his size, his Oldsmobile and pickup truck both had to be modified so the driver's seat could move back far enough to accommodate his long legs. Elsie Hartyl, Reid's receptionist for twenty years, recalled trying to drive the car with great difficulty; her legs were just too short.

❖❖❖

As the executive secretary of the Oregon Osteopathic Association for nearly thirty years, Reid was a faithful and effective voice for the osteopathic profession in Oregon. During that time, he was responsible for the organization of continuing medical education events, coordinating the meetings of the Board of Directors of the association, and serving to assist the succession of DOs who were association presidents. In short, he was the glue that held the association together.

Another task he undertook very effectively was to act as a lobbyist for the association when the state legislature was in session. He was a man of very strong convictions and it was not unusual for him to clash with those with whom he disagreed. Other DOs in the area recall that he would usually come to meetings a bit late, but with his booming voice, his opinions would always be heard. He worked very hard to pave the way for osteopathic physicians in the state to have full medical rights and privileges.

He also served for twenty years as the osteopathic representative on the Oregon State Board of Medical Examiners (now the Oregon Medical Board), interceding on behalf of some doctors and conscientiously working to protect Oregonians from misbehaving physicians.

Reid tried to retire once, but after nearly fifty years of practice and with 14,000 patients of record, he had developed a following of loyal and loving patients who simply wouldn't hear of him quitting. He did return to practice for a time, but he developed diplopia, a harbinger of lung cancer, to which he succumbed a few months later.

Despite the fact that he died thirty-one years ago, many of his patients remember this gentle giant very fondly. There is no doubt that the memory of his wonderful contributions to the community of Lebanon and to the osteopathic profession were instrumental in helping to prepare a warm and approving welcome to the new college of osteopathic medicine in Lebanon.

Arthur Rott, DO 1948 – 2012

I interviewed Dr. Arthur Rott and his wife Christi at their home in West Linn, Oregon. Rott, like some of the other osteopathic specialists who practiced at Eastmoreland Hospital, had a tremendous impact on the osteopathic profession throughout Oregon. Although he was a specialist in oncology, hematology, and internal medicine, his first love was always teaching. As a teacher, he touched the lives and careers of many of the osteopathic physicians who practice in Oregon and throughout the Northwest.

Rott took his premed education at Wayne State University in Detroit, Michigan. At the suggestion and advice of a friend, he applied to and was accepted at the Chicago College of Osteopathic Medicine in 1969. He had never lived far from home, so his years at Chicago were memorable. A rigorous educational program had been introduced at the school which required weekly exams in all subjects, covering current material as well as going back to the first week of classes. After Rott graduated, he had his pick of internships, ultimately settling for Zieger-Botsford Hospital in Detroit, Michigan. This 400-bed hospital was a wonderful training ground for young interns; however, his resident supervisor on nights told him that if he woke him during the night he would break his legs. It was clearly a sink-or-swim situation, and Rott thrived in every area except obstetrics. So he traded night call with the obstetrics resident, covering everything in the hospital except obstetrics.

During that busy time, Rott found time to date Christi Perry, whose deceased father, Charles Perry, was a Detroit police detective. They met on a blind date. They married in 1976, a marriage that has endured to this day. Four years later, the young couple had a son, Barry, who is now pursuing a career as an osteopathic physician.

Rott entered an internal medicine residency at Zieger-Botsford Hospital in Farmington Hills, Michigan, followed by a two-year fellowship in hematology/oncology at Martin Place Hospital in Madison Heights, Michigan. He completed his training in 1978 and immediately went into practice with one of his mentors, Harold Margolis, DO, in Madison Heights. His parents resided in Detroit and on only one occasion, medical school, had he ever gone very far from home.

There was one small problem—he was so busy with the practice that he had little time to devote to his new wife Christi or to outside activities. He had been in contact with his friend Arnie Miller, who had come to Portland as the first osteopathic hematologist/oncologist at Eastmoreland Hospital in Portland, Oregon. Miller assured him that specialists in Oregon weren't required to work long hours and the climate and surroundings were wonderful—it was great place to live and raise a son.

Little did Rott know that he had been lured into a very busy practice that not only included the responsibilities of a hematology/oncology practice but the day-to-day education of interns and medical students. His sense of humor, his gentle manner, and his humility made him an instant success as a teacher and mentor. The hospital staff loved him and, as a result, he was busier and had more responsibilities than ever.

Rott's dry sense of humor and fun manifested itself in the way he taught. He often reminded folks that he was the only osteopathic "triple-boarded" internist, hematologist, and oncologist in Oregon, probably in the entire Northwest. At the annual hospital Christmas party, his rendition of "The Dreidel Song" was famous. He rarely passed up a chance to have some fun, even if was at his own expense.

As a staff member of a small hospital, he had the usual responsibilities as chair of the medicine department. He was also a member and ultimately the chairman of the medical education committee, and later served as director of medical education. Rott played an important role in the development of the Family Practice Residency program at the hospital. He was also instrumental in the formation of the FamilyCare Insurance Plan and was its medical director until his retirement in 2006. He has been on the board of directors and chaired multiple organizations.

Rott has received several prestigious awards, including Educator of the Year on multiple occasions from the house staff at Eastmoreland Hospital, Charles Carlstrom DO Lecture Award from the Northwest Osteopathic Medical Foundation, DO of the Year award from Osteopathic Physicians of Oregon, J. Scott Heatherington Award from the Northwest Osteopathic Medical Foundation, and

Pumerantz Lifetime Fellow of Excellence in Osteopathic Medical Education from the College of Osteopathic Medicine, Western University, Pomona, California.

Portland Osteopathic Hospital, later Eastmoreland Hospital, has had a training program since it was founded in 1945. Each year, four to six osteopathic physicians graduated to either practice locally, go on to a residency program, or move to another state. When Rott arrived in 1978, he immediately began to teach interns and students and later residents. We showed him a list of doctors with whom he had had personal contact and trained over the years since his arrival. There were 137 residents and interns on the list; this does not include the many medical students who interacted with Rott over those years. Many of these doctors, including the dean of the COMP-Northwest, are leaders and practice with distinction in our community today. What a legacy.

Rott said the most difficult challenge he faced in his career was to be the spouse of a cancer patient and later as a cancer patient himself. His greatest satisfaction has been his career as a teacher and enjoying the friendship and admiration of his colleagues and students. A recent happy moment was when he had the thrill of placing a white coat on his son Barry as he embarked on his education as an osteopathic physician at COMP-Northwest.

Rott said the formation of the school in Lebanon, and the wholehearted support that project is receiving from the community and around the state, hold great promise for the continued success of the profession.

Bertha Sawyer, DO 1872 – 1974

Of the early osteopathic physicians who practiced in Oregon, Bertha Sawyer was the very first to practice in southern Oregon. Little is known about her early life except that she was born in Fairview, Kansas, on July 25, 1872, and she spent her formative years in northeastern Kansas. Her parents were Cyrus Alexander

Sawyer and Delia Frances Hull. She attended the Still College of Osteopathic Medicine in Des Moines, Iowa, graduating in 1901.

In 1902, she joined her sister in Klamath Falls and then moved to Ashland, where she began her osteopathic practice at 125 Oak Street in 1903. She quickly established herself in practice and joined the American Osteopathic Association. She also became active in the Oregon Osteopathic Association. In 1908, she and sixty-seven other DOs were issued their licenses by the Oregon Board of Medical Examiners.

Throughout the 1910s and 1920s, Sawyer seems to have changed office locations in Ashland frequently. In 1911, she had offices in the Rhodes-Fankow Building; in 1917, she moved to the Pioneer Building, and in 1919, she was practicing in the First National Bank Building. During that time she began to develop a bedside method for treating spleens with good results. Her original work was conducted at her sanitarium in Ashland, but the record is silent as to the particulars of the sanitarium.

DOs were barred from practicing in any allopathic hospitals at that time and were often forced to form their own infirmaries or sanitariums. Sawyer, in conjunction with an osteopathic husband-and-wife team, Drs. Jack and Gladys Crandall, held a series of clinics devoted to teaching her methods for treating splenic conditions along the West Coast and other parts of the country. T. J. Ruddy, a Los Angeles DO, published a travel journal in the *Western Osteopath* which documented this series of clinics. According to the 1930 census, she spent the remaining years of her career at 18 Main Street in Ashland. She may have had her office and residence connected at the time.

Sawyer was an avid collector of Native American artifacts, which she donated to the Southern Oregon College and Museum in Ashland. Some of her collection can also be found at the Southern Oregon Historical Society Library in Medford, Oregon.

She was very involved in community affairs, including Martha Gillette Guild, Daughters of the American Revolution, the Women's Civic Club of the Oregon Federation of Women's Clubs,

Hope Rebekah Lodge, and the Ashland Garden Club. She was an active member of First Presbyterian Church in Ashland. She continued to be an active member of the Oregon Osteopathic Association and the American Osteopathic Association throughout her career, and she was involved in the formation of the Southern Oregon Osteopathic Society.

Little is known about Sawyer's personal life; it is not known if she ever married. She retired from active practice in 1947 at the age of seventy-five, after forty-four years of practice. She was a well-known and beloved physician, a pillar of her community, and remained in Ashland for the remainder of her life. By her one-hundredth birthday, she was a resident at the Ashland Community Hospital. She died on January 10, 1974.

Howard Scalone, DO 1932 –

Many of the doctors that I have interviewed have such interesting and influential lives that our attempts to summarize their stories do not do them justice. Dr. Howard Scalone certainly fits in this category, with a truly amazing career that has yet to end.

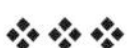

Scalone was born into a Italian family in the Bronx, New York. He was an only child, but his extended family included thirteen uncles and aunts. In the difficult economic times that followed the market crash of 1929, his father found work where he could. At an early age, Scalone was interested in becoming a doctor; when he was seven, he put out a shingle on the front of the family home announcing he was a veterinary doctor. When a woman came to the house seeking help for her ailing dog, Scalone's mother brought his career as a vet to an abrupt end.

At Cardinal High School, an all-boys Catholic school, Scalone enjoyed the sciences. He was a member of the student council and lettered for four years in track and cross country. Scalone applied to three colleges and decided to go with the first one that accepted him. This turned out to be Pomona College in Pomona, California, a school noted for its strong science emphasis. Scalone majored in a track called zoo/chem.

In July of 1952, between his second and third years at the school, he eloped with Josephine Korenkiewicz and they were married by a justice of the peace in New Hampshire. (He got married in New Hampshire because he was only twenty years old—too young to marry in New York without parental consent.)

He graduated in 1953 after three years of college. At the time, the tuition was a flat annual fee, so you could take twenty-one or twenty-two units for the price of fifteen. He was prompted to complete the degree in three years mostly as an economic measure. The Korean War was underway at this time, and many young men were drafted. To fulfill his obligation, Scalone joined ROTC and later transferred to the Navy Reserve as a corpsman.

While in college, he learned that his best friend was interested in osteopathic medicine and was applying to the Still College of Osteopathic Medicine in Des Moines, Iowa. Scalone was so impressed by his friend's experience that he also applied to Des Moines and was accepted for the class of 1958. At the time of Scalone's college graduation, the young couple was expecting their first child. Josephine wanted to have the baby in her hometown, so they moved to Connecticut to be close to family when the baby arrived.

From 1953 to 1954, Scalone worked for Dow Chemical as a chemist. In the summer of 1954, while living in New York, he met New York Supreme Court Justice Levi, who inquired as to their future plans. When Scalone informed him that they were going to the Des Moines school that fall, the judge asked why they were going so far. Scalone replied that it was the only school he had applied to. Judge Levi asked if he would like to go to the Philadelphia school. Scalone thought it was too late to apply, but Judge Levi advised him to apply anyway. Scalone was interviewed by the school, but he had not heard from them by the beginning of September, so he and Josephine packed their car and prepared to go to Des Moines.

Scalone decided to make a phone call to Philadelphia to ask about his application before they drove off. He was told he had been accepted, but Scalone had not received the acceptance letter. So they drove to Philadelphia instead of Des Moines.

The Philadelphia school was noted for its excellent osteopathic manipulation therapy and anatomy departments, both headed by Dr. Angus Kathie. Scalone did well in anatomy and soon became a teacher's assistant. He had been plagued for years by migraine headaches, and one day Kathie noted that Scalone was in pain. Right there in the lab, Kathie gave him a cranial therapy treatment; Scalone slept for three hours and never had a migraine again. (To this day Scalone uses OMT as a diagnostic tool and as a treatment.)

Scalone graduated in 1958, and was accepted that same year to a rotating internship at Garden City Hospital just outside of Detroit. The program was a true rotating internship where the interns learned by practice the many skills needed to be a successful DO general practitioner (GP).

After completing his internship in 1959, he took a position as a GP in small New York resort area called Mastic Beach, with a population of 3,000. An MD friend of Scalone's family gave him privileges in the local proprietary hospital, and he and two other doctors provided medical care to the people of the community.

Over the winter things were fairly calm, so Scalone did most of his own surgeries, made house calls, and performed other duties as needed. When summer came, the population swelled to 30,000. Suddenly he became very busy, seeing patients over long hours, with an average of twenty house calls and emergency room visits a day. He was also on call for the local police and called upon to pronounce death by drowning on several occasions. In his last few days at Mastic Beach, he averaged one delivery a day.

With a young family to raise, it became evident that this was too much, so he left and undertook a two-year residency in anesthesia at Garden Grove Hospital. His initial training was in the use of ether and cyclopropane.

After this residency, Scalone worked at various hospitals, including one in Florida, and ended up at Northwest Osteopathic Hospital in Milwaukee, Wisconsin. For the next seventeen years, Scalone worked at Northwest, where he was often called upon to do angiograms, myelograms, carotid artery studies, and other procedures not in the usual job description of an anesthesiologist. He also held senior obstetrical privileges because of his skill with forceps deliveries. He was chief of staff and held many other positions at Northwest, including director of medical education. He was also active in Wisconsin osteopathic politics and was appointed by the governor to the joint committee on medical education.

In May 1980, he and his wife decided to move to Oregon to be closer to his son David, who was having serious medical problems. When he applied for his Oregon license, he was interviewed by Robert Butler, DO, who suggested that he should apply to Eastmoreland Hospital to take the place of the retiring Dr. Burnham Brooke. At Eastmoreland, he practiced anesthesiology and started a pain clinic. He also was on staff at other hospitals where he was recognized and appreciated for his versatile skills.

To stave off boredom, he and his wife and family built their home outside of Vancouver, Washington. She drew up the plans and Scalone and his family constructed the home, which was uniquely designed to be energy efficient. He took up gardening, and in 2005, he was awarded a Master Gardener degree; he is also a certified beekeeper. In a more active vein, he sailed as crew of a boat to Hawaii and to the Fiji Islands.

One day a week he works in a free clinic in Vancouver, and is the "go-to guy" for folks who need OMT. He is often shadowed by medical students from Oregon Health and Science University. Recently, he was called upon by a local dentist and has been giving anesthesia to patients undergoing full-mouth procedures. He was also a valued member of the team that helped to interview and select the students at COMP-Northwest.

When asked about his greatest achievements, he said the first was marrying his wife, because of her wonderful support and participation in his practice over the years; the second was becoming a DO. His greatest disappointment was the death of his son at age thirty. He also was saddened by the loss of osteopathic hospitals across the country. His advice to prospective DOs: "Go for it!"

Sheridan Thiringer, DO 1936 –

The Maple Street Clinic in Forest Grove was the first osteopathic hospital to "spin off" from Portland Osteopathic Hospital. From the beginning, it was staffed by a remarkable group of DOs who served their community in numerous ways, including the formation of Forest Grove Hospital. One of the key physicians at that hospital and clinic was Sheridan "Sherry" Thiringer, DO.

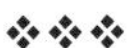

Thiringer was born and raised in Spokane, Washington. In high school he learned the shoe repair trade and later entered the iron working trade. After graduation, he enrolled at Gonzaga University in Spokane as a premed student, supporting himself as a shoe repairman in winter and as a bridge construction worker in summer. After high school, he had enlisted in the Navy reserve, and, since it was the Vietnam War era, he was required to join the Army ROTC. For a while he was in both services. During that time he also married his first wife.

Early on, Thiringer was determined to become an osteopathic physician, and throughout his premed education there was no doubt as to his goal. After graduation from Gonzaga in 1959, he was accepted to the Des Moines College of Osteopathic Medicine in 1959 and graduated in 1963.

Thiringer was determined to set up practice in the Northwest as close as possible to his home in Spokane. He was accepted as an intern at Portland Osteopathic Hospital in 1963. While interning he became interested in practicing internal medicine and hoped to serve under the mentorship of Robert Conley, DO, an internist at the hospital. After completing his internship in 1964, circumstances dictated that there would be a prolonged delay before he could begin his internal medicine fellowship. With a family to support, Thiringer began to search for practice opportunities to tide him over. He was contacted by T. M. Hobart, DO, who was searching for someone to help with his large and busy practice in Vernonia, Oregon.

Not long after Thiringer joined Hobart, Hobart left the practice, leaving Thiringer to cover this busy practice by himself. Thiringer practiced solo in Vernonia for two years. While practicing full time, he had to deal with some difficult personal family matters, and reluctantly decided to leave as well. He joined the fledgling Forest Grove Hospital staff and the Maple Street Clinic.

At the clinic, Thiringer served as a GP, but as the hospital became increasingly busy, it became evident that a second anesthesiologist was needed. After a few months of studying at Eastmoreland Hospital under Robert Butler, DO, he became the hospital's second anesthesiologist.

While practicing in Vernonia and later in Forest Grove, Thiringer became involved in the local communities. He was the team physician for Vernonia High School, and later Forest Grove High School. He was the team physician for all sports at Pacific University in Forest Grove, and deputy investigator/coroner for Washington County. During that time, he was often called to testify in court in sanity hearings. He was an educator of emergency medical technicians (EMTs) throughout Washington County, and acted as department physician for the Washington County sheriff's department. He also served as physician advisor to the Vernonia and Forest Grove fire departments. Later, because he was not board certified in anesthesiology, he stopped his practice as an anesthesiologist and joined the staff of Tuality Hospital in Hillsboro. Today, he still works one day at the Maple Street Clinic and as a consultant at the Tuality Hospital on the complexities of Medicare coding rules.

As a member of the staff of the small Forest Grove Hospital, he served on nearly every committee at one time or another. Later he served for six years on the Oregon Board of Medical Examiners and was responsible for supervising EMTs and paramedics licensed by the State of Oregon.

Early in his medical career, Thiringer rejoined the Navy as a commissioned officer in the reserves. This duty was more like a vacation, and one of the perks of the position was to serve as locum at various United States embassies around the world. He retired from the Navy Reserve as a captain at age sixty.

Thiringer and his two young children had to leave his first marriage. He acted as a single dad for several years while performing his many medical and community duties. When he was called to the hospital for emergency anesthesia, the children often accompanied him, sleeping in the doctor's dressing room and cared for by the RNs on the staff—including forays to the kitchen for midnight ice cream! Thiringer says that his son Kim can recall arriving on the scene of a fatal accident at night, blue lights flashing. The children were well known at the sheriff's office, the local fire station, and other locations around Forest Grove. Thiringer states he could not have done all the things that he did without the support of the people of the community. The people of Vernonia and Forest Grove became his family.

Today Thiringer lives with his second wife, Judy, on their farm in Vernonia, raising bees, chickens, and Kobe beef. His son Kim Thiringer, DO, is a practicing ENT specialist in Hillsboro, and his daughter Sherri resides with her family in the Midwest.

The greatest challenge of his life was balancing the duties of his profession and being a single parent. He says, "It has been an honor to be able to work in the osteopathic profession as a caring physician of service to humanity."

Frank Trostel, DO 1936 – 2013

One of the challenges that all medical organizations face is finding people who will step forward and volunteer for various committees, special tasks, meeting coordination, and so on. Further complicating the challenge is that a person who does volunteer may fail to perform; those who do volunteer and perform well are in the minority. Dr. Frank Trostel was one who frequently volunteered, and when he did so, leadership could rely on the fact that the job would be done and done well.

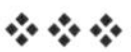

Trostel was born in 1936 in St. Joe, Indiana, and his earliest recollections of the medical care he received was from a local osteopathic physician, Dr. Dale Treadwell. Trostel so admired Treadwell that he decided at an early age to become a DO himself. After premed at Manchester College in Manchester, Indiana, he enrolled in the same osteopathic school where Treadwell received his training, Chicago College of Osteopathic Medicine. Trostel recalled the school had a rigorous academic and clinical regime that assured students of the most up-to-date and best possible education in osteopathic medicine.

After his second year, Trostel had a ten-week hiatus during which he was allowed to select his own externship. He, along with fellow student Rolland Schultheis, opted for a rotation at Portland Osteopathic Hospital. Neither of the young students had been to either coast, so when they received an offer to come to Portland and were offered a travel allowance of $50 and a stipend of $25 per week plus room and board, they leaped at the chance. Trostel said that for the first time he was treated as a doctor. Upon their graduation in 1961, both the young DOs came to Portland for their internships.

The internship year was an eventful one for Trostel. Early on, he exhibited the characteristics that would mark him for leadership roles later in his career. He states that his knowledge of Robert's Rules of Order and an understanding of the hospital bylaws caused him to speak up at staff meetings, often challenging motions that were not permitted in the bylaws.

As an intern, he also exhibited a competence and confidence that made him a prime prospect for doctors who were seeking associates. One such DO, Al Greenway, had recently arrived from the Chicago school, where he was director of the clinics. Greenway invited Trostel to join him, and the two doctors opened a clinic in Portland in September 1962.

Almost from the start, the clinic was a success. Both doctors worked five days a week and did their own obstetrics. They did their hospital rounds in the early morning, and then worked at their clinic from 9 a.m. until 6 p.m.; they were on-call every other week. Things were going smoothly until the sudden and unexpected death of Greenway. After Greenway's death, Trostel struggled to accommodate all of the patients he had suddenly inherited in addition to his own practice. For a time, Robert Todd, DO, joined him, but he departed for Tillamook, Oregon, leaving Trostel with even more patients.

While running his busy practice, which included forty deliveries a year, Trostel also began to take on hospital responsibilities. Less than a year into practice, he was on the Medical Audit Committee. Following this, he served on virtually every hospital committee, often as chairman, also serving as chief of staff for a term.

Because he was doing such a good job, he was recommended to the Oregon Osteopathic Association, where he came under the mentoring of Dave Reed, DO. Reed was secretary/treasurer of the association and represented the osteopathic profession on the State Board of Medical Examiners. Reed asked Trostel to be program chairman of the annual continuing education committee. From 1967 to 1972, Trostel acted as executive director of the Oregon Osteopathic Association. Trostel was appointed by Governor McCall as the alternate member of the Oregon Board of Medical Examiners, and he also served on the Multnomah Foundation for Medical Care, Oregon Medical Practice Review Board, Oregon Medical Practice PAC, and other committees.

In 1975, after the abrupt departure of the hospital administrator, Kip Castle, Trostel found himself volunteering to be acting administrator of the hospital. He rearranged his office schedule so that he saw patients in his office from 6:30 a.m. until noon, and then came to the hospital after lunch. He states that it was probably the most challenging two years of his career. He had no experience dealing with labor unions, yet he was called upon to deal with a unionization movement (which failed), the dismissal of an intern, political squabbling among staff members, and a host of other challenges. Two years later, he was asked to continue as the administrator, but at that point he said he had to quit. However, he continued to hold responsible positions at the hospital for five years, including medical director.

While representing the Oregon Osteopathic Association on a national level, he and Jerry Lancaster, DO, were instrumental in organizing a group called the Small States Group, which voted as a block to fend off the political maneuvers of states with large DO concentrations. One such motion was to expel every DO in Oregon and Washington who joined MD organizations to obtain malpractice insurance. (This motion was defeated.)

Even in the midst of his busy professional career, Trostel somehow found the time to pursue his hobby of flying. In short order, he was a member of the Civil Air Patrol (CAP), served as this organization's medical officer from 1966 to 1968, then served as commander of Oregon Senior Pilots Squadron. He received the National CAP Citation for his outstanding service to the Civil Air Patrol.

In 1996, Trostel retired and moved to Bend, Oregon. Soon it became evident that he wasn't quite ready to retire, so he took a position at a struggling clinic in Sisters, Oregon. What he offered to the patients was the services of an experienced and caring osteopathic physician. To better serve the community, he offered free sports physicals for children, which caused consternation among the MDs practicing in the area. When a newspaper ad appeared in the local paper claiming that the MD mentioned was the best trained doctor in the community, Trostel stated that this got his "competitive juices flowing!" Needless to say, the practice prospered.

Trostel retired for the second time in 2001. He and his wife Arista reside near Bend. Despite being retired, Trostel maintains a lively interest in the community and in the osteopathic profession. He is very excited about COMP-Northwest and plans to support that effort in any way he can.

His greatest satisfaction has been in volunteering to serve in so many capacities and completing those tasks successfully. His greatest disappointment was the closure of Eastmoreland Hospital.

His advice to incoming students: "Learn all you can and when opportunity arises, volunteer and be an asset to your profession and the community you will serve."

Al Turner, DO 1944 –

All osteopathic physicians receive instruction in osteopathic manipulation, also known as osteopathic manual therapy (OMT), as part of their training curriculum. In earlier times, this skill was the primary tool used by the DO. Today, because of time constraints and poor reimbursement by third parties, the average DO rarely uses OMT, relying on medical treatments for the preponderance of their patients. This is the story of a DO who started his practice as a primary care physician using mostly medical treatments, but who evolved to become a true osteopathic physician whose philosophy is very close to the original precepts taught by A. T. Still.

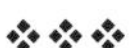

Turner was born in Monett, Missouri, the youngest son of a railway clerk who invented the ZIP code system used by the U.S. Postal Service. His mother was primarily a homemaker and a devout Free Methodist; it was her fondest wish that one of her children be a missionary, and since Turner was the youngest child, he was elected.

At age eight, Turner and his family moved to Kansas. Turner attended a small high school where he excelled in academics and sports. His six-foot, four-inch frame was perfect for basketball. He was on the honor roll, performed in the class play, and had a role in student government. He continued to be active in the local Free Methodist Church as well.

After graduating from high school in 1962, he enrolled in Central College in McPherson, Kansas. After two years, he transferred to

Spring Arbor College, graduating in 1967. He entered seminary with the aim of sharpening his ministerial skills, but the curriculum of the school was actually designed to give students only the concepts of ministry. He left the seminary after a quarter.

At the time, the Vietnam War was in full swing, and the draft was a constant threat. With his background and religious training, he was adamantly opposed to killing and applied for conscientious objector status. After some wrangling, the draft board labeled him an "objector of conscience" and required him to serve for two years as a counselor at a school for "emotionally disturbed, socially maladjusted, delinquent juvenile males." During this time, Turner determined that he needed more training as a teacher and counselor, so after he completed his time at the school, he enrolled in the master's in counseling program at Western Michigan University in Kalamazoo. After graduation and the receipt of his master's degree, Turner served as Coordinator of Religious Affairs at the university.

Since the age of five, Turner had wanted to be a physician, specifically a missionary doctor, but when he flunked chemistry, he believed that career was forever closed to him. While working at Western Michigan University, he applied to the University of Michigan medical school and was advised that at twenty-eight years old, he was too old to be accepted. A premed counselor at Western advised him that he might be better suited as an osteopathic physician, a profession that he knew nothing about.

In 1972, Turner injured his back pushing cars during a blizzard. Because of severe back spasms, he sought treatment from a local MD who prescribed pain pills and advised him to rest. For two weeks, he was unable to walk upright; in desperation, he sought treatment from a local DO. After one treatment, he was able to walk upright and soon was back to his old self. This convinced Turner that osteopathic medicine was the career he must follow.

He was accepted into the Michigan State University College of Osteopathic Medicine in 1974, graduating in 1978. While at the college, he was trained by some of the leading practitioners of

OMT in the country. He said he felt that he was being trained by the "cream of the crop" all the way through his four years. (He has written an interesting essay in which he discusses the mentors who influenced him during those years and later in practice.)

While he was growing up, Turner's family would leave Kansas during the summer and go to Oregon, where they resided with an aunt and harvested cherries and other crops to raise money for the "vacation" and school clothes. Turner fell in love with the area and determined that sometime in his life he would make it his home. So when the opportunity arose for an internship at Eastmoreland Hospital in Portland, he took it, graduating in 1979.

After the internship, Turner started his career in Salem, Oregon, but for various reasons left that practice and took over the practice of Dr. Robert Woodmansee, a DO in Hillsboro, Oregon. After a time, he managed to transform this practice into a success, but became bored with the routine. At an AOA convention in Chicago, he was recruited by the West Virginia College of Osteopathic Medicine to be the medical director at a State of West Virginia hospital and clinic in a small coal-mining town called Welch. He quickly discovered that the staff consisted of four doctors, two medical students, and two RNs. It was his job to bring the place up to speed so that when a 120-bed replacement hospital and clinic were built, the staff would be well prepared.

After one year in this gloomy, unrewarding environment, he relocated to Florida where there was lots of sunshine. For the first six years of his twelve years in Florida, he was medical director of a chain of urgent care centers. The last six years he worked as a primary care doctor in a small clinic where he could use more and more of his OMT skills.

In 1993, he answered an advertisement for director of the OMT Department at Eastmoreland Hospital in Portland, Oregon. He got the job and continued in that position until the closure of the hospital in 2004. Following this, he set up a private practice in nearby Johns Landing called Osteopathic Advantage Clinic, which was devoted exclusively to OMT. He continued to practice in that location until his retirement in June 2013.

Throughout his career, Turner has been involved in training future osteopathic physicians as a lecturer and as a mentor. His training positions include Graduate Teaching Fellow, Michigan State University of Osteopathic Medicine; Adjunct Associate Clinical Professor, Osteopathic Medicine, Touro Osteopathic, Vallejo, California; Clinical Faculty, Midwestern University, Arizona College of Osteopathic Medicine, Glendale, Arizona; Clinical Professor of OMT Western University of Health Sciences, Pomona, California; Associate Professor of Family Medicine, West Virginia College of Osteopathic Medicine, Lewisburg, West Virginia; Associate Professor of Osteopathic Medicine, A. T. Still School of Osteopathic Medicine, Mesa, Arizona; and Clinical Associate Professor, Department of Family Medicine, Oregon Health and Science University. He also teaches a course on osteopathic medicine at Portland State University each year.

Turner has been involved in a host of community organizations too numerous to list. Most notable was his recent election as president of the Multnomah County Medical Society. He has also been involved in Osteopathic Physicians and Surgeons of Oregon (OPSO) as a board member. He has been the recipient of numerous awards and recognitions due to his many contributions to the osteopathic profession.

To the many students and residents who have had the privilege of working with Turner in his office or in the clinics, his greatest contribution to the profession has been his ability to teach. As a mentor, he has been honored on many occasions, including a 2013 award recognizing his contribution to the educational program at COMP-Northwest.

In addition to his practice and mentoring, Turner served as a volunteer minister, preacher, missionary, and medical student mentor in Peru, Haiti, Jamaica, Mexico, and Ireland. His advice to those who wish to go on mission trips: "Don't consider going unless you are prepared to have your heart broken and your life changed forever. The bad news is that you will never again see the world through the eyes of innocence; your life will be changed forever. The good news is that the heart must be broken in order to expand."

Turner is married with two stepchildren and eight grandchildren. His wife Beryl, an accomplished woman in her own right, is a retired math and science teacher. Her support and advice have been very important in enabling Turner to be so active and involved.

Turner's most satisfying accomplishment has been to teach; to "see the lights come on in both patients and students" as they discover the "osteopathic advantage."

Birdie Eugenie Willis, DO 1925 –

Dr. Birdie Eugenie Willis, "Genie" to her friends, came to Oregon and the osteopathic profession in a manner that can only be described as "the hard way." Still very energetic despite her years, she speaks her mind and she has been an example and an inspiration to the young DO students she has trained, and especially to the young women who have entered the profession. At her request, her story is told in her own words, as they were related to me.

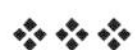

I was born in the prairie town of Bengough, Saskatchewan, and spent my early years in the little village of Ritchie where my father sold oil during the developing machine age and my mother was the local postmistress. I was the middle of three children—I had an older sister, Marguerite, and a younger brother, Bob. From the age of six, I attended a small one-room country school in Rexall.

I knew and had high regard for Dr. Ireland, who rode the circuit for the area on horseback or using a democrat (sleigh). He always stopped for Mom's coffee and had time to talk to me. My enjoyment of his conversation and company resulted in me telling him I wanted to be a doctor just like him. He encouraged the idea, and emboldened by this, I asked if I could have the next baby he found in his black bag. He answered yes! Much to my chagrin, he gave the next one to Mrs. Scott, and this made my list of disappointments. It took him a long time to find out what had happened to our relationship, but he eventually did. We had a long discussion and were once again best friends. Somehow, the idea of becoming a doctor stuck with me.

At age eight, I witnessed firsthand the drought that created the Dust Bowl in the prairies of the United States and Canada. It was no longer possible to grow a garden, which had been a staple and a source of fresh vegetables for the family. The Great Depression arrived. My family was in the process of building our home, but the Bank of Weyburn went bankrupt, so we moved to Ogema and a farm belonging to my Great-uncle Joseph. Winter was close at hand, and we were glad to have a warm house.

I was in high school in WWII, and in 1943, during my junior year, I quit school and joined the Canadian Women's Army Corps. I served on the Headquarters Staff with the Provost Corps and G2 Intelligence. At the end of the conflict, I continued in the Reserve Force, attaining the rank of Captain. I am still a Canadian citizen and a "green card carrier," renewing as necessary.

After the war, I held many jobs, including teaching at Reliance School of Commerce, selling advertising in Fraser's Canadian Trade Directories, selling printing supplies, and finally working as the secretary to the business manager of the Camsell Indian Tuberculosis Hospital in Edmondton, Alberta. The "doctor bug" bit again. I was able to use my military credits to return to a pre-matriculation school in Calgary, so now I could start university training. However, there was still a point system for university admission to give the male veterans priority, so I went back to work for another hospital administrator, then back to teaching at Hendersons Secretarial School. In a few months, I learned I was turning out students who were earning more than I was. So it was back to the drawing board once more.

I then moved to Windsor, Ontario, and was employed as a secretary with the city solicitor. The United States was just across the Detroit River, and I became a "nickel immigrant." (A nickel was the price of a bus ride across the border to Detroit). Hygrade Food Products and Bigelow Liptak Corporation were employers who expanded my horizons. The engineering firm used my services to organize their construction department. I supervised two installations I take a lot of pride in: Shell Oil in Anacortes, Washington, and ARAMCO in Saudi Arabia.

These projects were exciting and fulfilling until I found out it was possible to obtain a university degree by attending night school. Eight years later, with my BA/Sc degree firmly in hand, I entered Chicago College of Osteopathy in Illinois. After my graduation in 1968, I headed west to Portland, Oregon. Dr. Paula Eschtruth had invited me to visit in December. It snowed while I was in Portland, and they were playing golf in the snow with red golf balls. What could be more inviting!

The internship at Portland Osteopathic Hospital with fellow Canadians Melvin Gerber, James Bondurant, and Michael Kozak was a lively year with the usual frustrations and excitement. The year 1969, the final step in a very long road with many turns and twists, was nearly complete. Where to hang my shingle?

A realtor in the area of Woodstock offered to sell me his office, an ideal situation. I had made a commitment to work alternate nights and weekends in the emergency room at the Eastmoreland Hospital to provide some cash flow until the patients found me and I could refer from the ER to my office. This situation continued for two years until I found a secretary who stayed with me for twenty-nine years. I was finally a general practitioner like Dr. Ireland, just as I had dreamed. As part of my hospital staff privileges, I served a term as chairman of the Intern Training Committee.

No one was ever refused service, and I gave full service to the best of my ability. I delivered babies, assisted in surgery, performed surgery, held hands (and slapped them when necessary), and was available to my patients twenty-four/seven until 2004.

At age seventy-nine, I thought it was time to try something new because there was a monumental change taking place in doctor/patient relationships. I was developing an interest in plants and gardening, so the next thing was bees. I particularly enjoy working with them and harvesting the fruits of their labors.

I missed the personal contact with my patients, so I charged into community activities. I joined and am still an active Rotarian. I also joined the local Neighborhood Association, Business Association, two garden clubs, a bridge club, and a pinochle club.

One of the saddest times for me was when Eastmoreland Hospital was sold and demolished. It hurts each time I drive by. The funds from the sale were invested in the Northwest Osteopathic Medical Association and funds and donations are now available for deserving DOs in training. I am pleased to support the females in any way I can. They just have to go for it!

The bright note on our horizon is the establishment of our own osteopathic university in Lebanon, Oregon, with the assistance of the College of Osteopathic Medicine of the Pacific from Pomona, California.

John F. Wood, DO 1923 – 2007

Driving west on Highway 26, "The Sunset Highway," from Portland, you will see the rich farmlands of the upper Tualatin Valley, a beautiful and verdant area. Slightly to the south are small little towns surrounded by berry farms, vineyards, and dairy farms. Nestled in the midst of this area just east of the foothills of the Coast Range is the little town of Forest Grove, the home of Pacific University. It is also the home of the Forest Grove Hospital and Maple Street Clinic, both of which were inspired and developed by a remarkable osteopathic physician, Dr. John Wood. (This brief biography is based on information included in Wood's unpublished autobiography; this was made available to me in March 2011 by his son Steve Wood).

❖❖❖

Wood was born in Sugar City, Colorado, where he spent the first eleven years of his life. His family faced the harsh winters, dry summers, and isolation as they attempted to make a living in that bleak area of eastern Colorado. He attended a one-room school with eleven other students, but when his father moved the family to Derby, California, he discovered that he was academically far ahead of the other students in his new school. His father found work in the booming oil fields of Taft, California, and there the family settled, allowing young Wood to attend Taft High School. While still in high school, Wood went to work in the oilfields himself in order to accumulate money for college tuition.

After his high school graduation at age sixteen, Wood hitch-hiked to Oregon. That summer he spent time with an old family friend, fishing and hunting and later working the bean fields. That was the time when he made up his mind that he would make Oregon his home.

His college days began at Taft Junior College in 1939. He had a lot of fun but soon discovered that his grades were suffering, though he did turn out for boxing, earning his golden gloves. He also participated as a cheerleader, which entitled him to a letter sweater. To earn money for his college education, he began to work at a local mortuary and for a time considered this as a career.

His "wake up call" came when he failed a course in economics and sought the advice of a career counselor. He told the counselor that he wanted to be a doctor but couldn't afford the tuition. The counselor advised him that there were resources to help him through medical school if that was what he wanted. In his unpublished autobiography, he recalled this as "the most important thirty minutes of my life."

After a rigorous summer of hard labor, Wood had accumulated enough money to enroll in Fresno State College. He had far more success academically, and he became eligible to apply to the California College of Osteopathic Medicine in Los Angeles. He assumed that his letter of acceptance to medical school would give him a deferral from the draft, but this was not the case. When he reported for the draft, he failed the physical due to color blindness, but he was drafted in spite of this. He was ordered to report to Fort McArthur at San Pedro, California, for induction on November 19, 1942.

After many months of basic and then advanced training, his unit, the Black Hawk Division, was shipped to Europe just in time to participate in the Battle of the Bulge, and then to serve with General Patton as the army advanced into Germany. This was in the early months of 1945. Wood has photos of himself and his buddies at the Eagle's Nest, Hitler's famous retreat. He made it through this campaign in one piece, but after a brief period, the Black Hawk Division was transferred from Germany to the Philippines in anticipation of a ground war on mainland Japan. In May 1946, he was discharged as a sergeant and awarded a Bronze Star and ribbons for his service. (His son Steve still has many of his father's war trophies, including battle swords and even a human skull.)

He married his sweetheart Helen Garrison on May 11, 1946, and later that same year enrolled in the osteopathic college in Los Angeles. He described his four-year stint as a "blur," but still found the time to be class president and to be active in a local church where he was superintendent of the Sunday school. In his autobiography, Wood states that his years in the army and as a boxer were good preparation for leadership. During that time, he became friends with a resident in neurology, Sam Sheppard, whose life became the basis of the TV series *The Fugitive*. He was a staunch supporter of Sheppard and was convinced of his innocence.

He graduated from medical school in June 1950, and completed a rotating internship at the Los Angeles Osteopathic Hospital, located right next to the 4,000-bed Los Angeles County Hospital. While there, he exhibited an aptitude for both neurology and obstetrics and gynecology. He was offered a residency in either, but he opted instead to get to work. The Woods moved north in their Studebaker automobile and joined Fred Richards, DO, in practice in Forest Grove, Oregon.

Soon the practice was flourishing and the doctors were traveling back and forth to the Portland Osteopathic Hospital to manage care for their patients. Wood and his wife joined a local church and quickly became vital active members, teaching Sunday school and joining in other church activities. Wood also joined the local Rotary club and served in many capacities in that organization. He was also active in scouting, and as a veteran, joined the VFW (the Forest Grove unit bears the name John Wood as its unit name). He served as president of the Oregon Osteopathic Association, and, in conjunction with Scott Heatherington, DO, worked hard to educate the state representatives about the osteopathic profession and what it had to offer to the people of Oregon.

In 1959, it became evident that the old building housing Portland Osteopathic Hospital was inadequate. The board acquired property and began to build the new hospital, named Eastmoreland Hospital, on the other side of the Willamette River. Wood and his associates felt this new location was too much of a drive from their medical office location, so they decided that they should build their own hospital in Forest Grove. The hospital founders were Wood, Dr. Fred Richards, and Dr. Verne Jackson. Each doctor had his own area of specialization: Wood's was obstetrics. To further that goal, he took a one-year residency in high-risk obstetrics under the tutelage of Dr. Richard Eby in Pomona, California.

While training, he began to use a vacuum extraction device introduced from Sweden. This device was a major improvement over forceps in extracting babies during difficult delivery situations, but it had one drawback: It left a very obvious—transient but nevertheless alarming—spot on the neonate head resembling a large toadstool with hair on top.

Wood liked to work out at a local YMCA, and in the steam room of that facility he met an engineer whose specialty was molding plastics. The two collaborated to create the plastic Mityvac extractor cup which was even more effective and did not leave "hairy toadstools" on the scalps of newborns. This device was a major hit with obstetricians and is now in use all over the world. (Interestingly, the device was used in space by the astronauts—though apparently not for obstetrical use!)

Wood was an innovator in the field of obstetrics. In addition to the extraction device, he also pioneered the concept of a "birthing center" in Oregon. At the time, there was an increasing dissatisfaction with the method of delivery all across the United States. In accepted practice, the mother came to the hospital in labor. There she was separated from the father and family and taken to a delivery room where she was put in stirrups, sedated, and so forth, until she gave birth. The result was often a groggy baby and a mother with various injuries. Added to this was the risk of staph infections, which were the bane of the obstetrics department. To counter this, more and more women were delivering their babies at home, often ending up in the emergency room with bleeding or other complications.

After studying obstetrics programs in other parts of the world, Wood began to incorporate ideas gleaned from his studies into his own practice. He then proposed a radical idea. The demand was for "home delivery," so why not have a "home delivery" in *his* home, the hospital. With the help of the RNs at the hospital and the support of the hospital staff, they designed a room that was as "homey" as possible. There was home-like furniture, soft music, even a bed for the father to sleep in so he could be at the side of the delivering mother. In this relaxed setting, the deliveries went smoothly, often with the assistance of the father, and usually the mom and baby went home the next day—far sooner than at other hospitals. As an additional bonus, the infection rate was far lower than other hospitals in the area. It was the first birthing center in Oregon; over five hundred babies a year were delivered there. Wood also trained and employed nurse midwives at the birthing center.

From its start in June 1964, the Forest Grove hospital was a success. Demand for services such as surgery and obstetrics increased, but from the very start, like so many small hospitals, Forest Grove Hospital did not have the strong financial support required by these institutions. By 1984, health maintenance organizations (HMOs) and preferred provider organizations (PPOs) began to emerge, forcing patients away from the small hospitals. Tuality Hospital made an offer to purchase the Forest Grove Hospital, and the offer was accepted by the Forest Grove Hospital board. One of the first departments to go was the obstetrics department.

Today, the Forest Grove Hospital structure still stands and is being used for medically related purposes. The Maple Street Clinic next door is still staffed by DOs.

Wood retired December 31, 1988. After his retirement, he continued to be involved in his church and community. With his son Steve, Wood developed an artesian well on his property into a source for bottled water that is still in use.

Wood died November 25, 2007. He was proud to be an osteopathic physician, and his contributions to the field of obstetrics and to the osteopathic profession will serve as an inspiration for generations to come. He often cited the saying, "The measure of a man's success is how much he helps others succeed."

Bibliography

Atwood, Kay. *An Honorable History.* Medford, Oregon: Grandee Printing Center, Inc., 1985

Bal, B. Sonny, MD, MBA. *An Introduction to Medical Malpractice in the United States,* Department of Orthopedic Surgery, University of Missouri-Columbia MC213 DC053.00

Foley, Dirk. "The Northwest Track Origins," *COMP-Northwesterly* (magazine of the College of Osteopathic Medicine of the Pacific), Volume 1, Issue 3, Spring 2014

Gant, Lois, ed. *One Hundred Years of Osteopathic Medicine: A Photographic History.* Greenwich Connecticut: Greenwich Press,1995

Gevitz, Norman. *The DOs.* Baltimore, Maryland: The Johns Hopkins Press, 2004

Ho, Robert W. H., DO, *Bones Out of Place?* Baltimore, Maryland: Noble House, 2003

Lynch, Vera Martin. *Free Land for Free Men.* Portland, Oregon: Artline Printing Inc., 1973

O'Hara, Marjorie. *Southern Oregon: Short Trips into History*. Jacksonville, Oregon: Southern Oregon Historical Society, 1985

Quinn, Thomas A. *The Feminine Touch*. Kirksville, Missouri: Truman State University Press, 2011

Robbins, William. *Landscapes of Promise: The Oregon Story*. Seattle, Washington: University of Washington Press, 1997

Seffinger, Michael A. *Resurgence: The Rebirth of Osteopathic Medicine in California*. Novi, Michigan: Samjill Publishing Company, 2011

Siefer, Ellis, DO, *A Proud History*. Alexandria, Virginia: Global Printing Inc., 1995

Still, Andrew Taylor. *Early Osteopathy in the Words of A. T. Still*, Robert V. Schnucker, ed. Kirksville, Missouri: The Thomas Jefferson University Press at Northeast Missouri State University, 1991

Sutherland Society, "General Information on Cranial Osteopathy," http://www.cranial.co.uk/page2.html

Varon, Jodi. "Ing Hay ("Doc Hay") (1862–1952)," *The Oregon Encyclopedia*, http://www.ohs.org

Wikipedia, "Muscle energy technique," last modified November 26, 2014, http://en.wikipedia.org/wiki/Muscle_energy_technique

Wikipedia, "Osteopathic manipulative medicine," last modified on September 28, 2014, http://en.wikipedia.org/wiki/Osteopathic_manipulative_medicine

Acknowledgements

Clearly a book like this would not be possible without the support and advice of a number of people.

Special thanks to my dear wife, Meredith, for her patience as I worked on this, my first book.

I would like to compliment the wonderful work of Norman Gevitz, PhD, and the superb documentation and research in his book, *The DOs.*

Thanks to the retired DOs and their families and friends who took the time for the personal interviews included in this book.

Special thanks to Charles Kaluza who encouraged me and gave excellent advice on how to publish this work.

Thanks to my editor, Diane Johnson of PageCraft, as she patiently educated me in the usage of Microsoft Word, and advised and revised until the final book was ready.

And thanks, of course, to Dean Paula Crone for writing the Foreword.

Finally, thank you to my friends and relatives for patiently listening to me talk about my passion for osteopathic history.

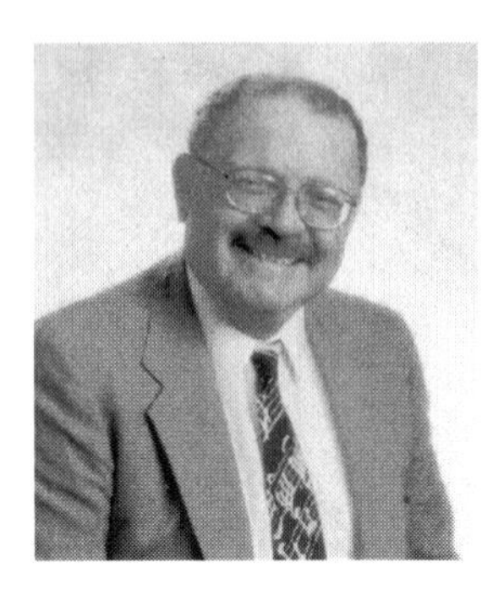

About the Author

John Stiger, DO, is a 1973 graduate of the Chicago College of Osteopathic Medicine. After a one-year rotating internship at Eastmoreland General Hospital in Portland, Oregon, Stiger practiced with Dr. John Bauers and others in Oak Grove, Oregon. He has served in many capacities on behalf of Eastmoreland Hospital and the profession in the state, including a six-year term on the Oregon Medical Board.

After retiring in 2008, he continues to practice osteopathic medicine at a free clinic in Oregon City, and assists as needed at the new osteopathic medical school in Lebanon, Oregon. He is an honorary member of the Advancement Board of the College of Osteopathic Medicine Northwest and was recently elected to the Board of Directors of the Northwest Osteopathic Medical Foundation.

Stiger is an avid reader and has also been writing biographies about fellow retired DOs since his own retirement. He and wife Meredith enjoy travel and are members of the Rolling Hills Community Church. He has three children and four grandchildren.

As an active member of the Rose City Garden Railroad Society, he enjoys creating miniature railroad structures in his shop. He and several other members open their layouts to the public every Father's Day.